The Moral Economy of AIDS i

Relatively few people have access to antiretroviral treatment in South Africa. The government justifies this on grounds of affordability. Nicoli Nattrass argues that the government's view insulates AIDS policy from social discussion and efforts to fund large-scale intervention.

Nattrass addresses South Africa's contentious AIDS policy from both an economic and ethical perspective, presenting:

- a history of AIDS policy in South Africa
- an expert analysis of the macroeconomic impact of AIDS
- a delineation of the relationship between AIDS and poverty and the challenges this poses for development, inequality and social solidarity
- an investigation into how a programme preventing mother-to-child transmission would be less expensive than having to treat children with AIDS-related illnesses
- an exploration of the relationship between AIDS treatment and risky sexual behaviour
- an economic and social case for expanded AIDS prevention and treatment intervention.

This relevant and accessible work is a valuable resource for readers with an interest in AIDS policy and the social and economic implications of the pandemic.

Nicoli Nattrass is Professor of Economics and Director of the Centre for Social Science Research at the University of Cape Town. Her research interests include economic policy, unemployment, inequality and AIDS in South Africa.

The Moral Economy of AIDS in South Africa

Nicoli Nattrass

*School of Economics and the
Centre for Social Science Research
University of Cape Town*

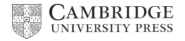

CAMBRIDGE
UNIVERSITY PRESS

CAMBRIDGE UNIVERSITY PRESS
Cambridge, New York, Melbourne, Madrid, Cape Town, Singapore, São Paulo

Cambridge University Press
The Water Club, Beach Road, Granger Bay, Cape Town 8005, South Africa

http://www.cambridge.org
Information on this title: www.cambridge.org/9780521548649

First published 2004
Reprinted 2006

Printed in South Africa by Creda Communications

Edited by Douglas van der Horst
Proof-reading by Tessa Kennedy
Cover artwork by Bulelwa Nokwe (left bodymap) and anonymous
(right bodymap)
Cover design by Karen Ahlschläger
Typeset by Vanessa Wilson in Utopia 10/13pt

ISBN-13   978-0-521-54864-9 paperback
ISBN-10   0-521-54864-0 paperback

Contents

For all those children who were born HIV-positive because the South African government said it could not afford to prevent mother-to-child transmission. It is also for the doctors, nurses and families who watched in anger and helplessness as more resources were spent coping with the children's AIDS-related illnesses than were needed to save them in the first place.

Acknowledgements

Special thanks to Jeremy Seekings for helping me sharpen my arguments during many long dog-walks on the mountain. I am particularly grateful to Jeremy, Sean Archer, David Benatar, Sean Muller, Evan Lieberman and Alan Whiteside for their critical and constructive reading of the manuscript.

I would also like to thank the following people for their comments and advice: Faried Abdullah, Frikkie Booysen, Andrew Boulle, Mike Cherry, Nathan Geffen, Alison Hickey, Leigh Johnson, Tony Leiman, Shannon Mitchell, Rinette van Coller and Desiré Vencatachellum. Celeste Coetzee and Vicki Elliott were very helpful research assistants.

I am grateful to Rob Dorrington and Leigh Johnson for allowing me to use the output of the ASSA2000 Interventions Model. I am grateful to the Andrew W. Mellon Foundation for providing me with teaching relief to complete the manuscript, and to SANPAD for their financial support of the project.

All financial proceeds from the book will go to the AIDS and Society Research Unit at the University of Cape Town.

Abbreviations

Acquired human immunodeficiency syndrome	AIDS
African National Congress	ANC
Antiretroviral	ARV
Actuarial Society of South Africa	ASSA
Zidovudine	AZT
Basic income grant	BIG
Centre for Actuarial Research	CARE
Computational general equilibrium	CGE
Congress of South African Trade Unions	COSATU
Directly observed therapy	DOT
Financial and Fiscal Commission	FFC
Growth, employment and redistribution	GEAR
Highly active antiretroviral therapy	HAART
Human immunodeficiency virus	HIV
Joint Health and Treasury Task Team	JHTTT
Medicines Control Council	MCC
Member of the executive committee [of a provincial government]	MEC
Medécins Sans Frontières	MSF
Men who have sex with men	MSM
Mother-to-child transmission prevention	MTCTP
Medium-term expenditure framework	MTEF
National AIDS Committee of South Africa	NACOSA
National Economic Development and Labour Council	NEDLAC
New Partnership for Africa's Development	NEPAD
Non-governmental organisation	NGO
Non-nucleoside reverse transcriptase inhibitor	NNRTI
Nucleoside analogue reverse transcriptase inhibitor	NRTI
Pharmaceutical Manufacturers' Association	PMA
Public works programme	PWP
Social accounting matrix	SAM
South African National AIDS Council	SANAC
Sexually transmitted disease	STD
Treatment Action Campaign	TAC
Unprotected anal intercourse	UAI
Value added tax	VAT
Voluntary counselling and testing	VCT

Figures

Tables

1 Introduction

The AIDS pandemic in Southern Africa is not only a major public health crisis but also a threat to economic development and social solidarity. South Africa, which is home to more HIV-positive people than any other country in the world, is a particularly interesting case in point. More than one in five adult South Africans are HIV-positive and AIDS deaths are expected to rise sharply until 2010. Over a million children could be orphaned by 2015 as a result. Such health shocks are devastating, not only for families and communities but also for the broader society and economy.

In August 2003, after many years of resistance and prevarication, the South African government finally bowed to public pressure and announced its support in principle for public-sector provision of highly active antiretroviral therapy (HAART). If offered rapidly and on a large enough scale, this has the potential to ameliorate the impact of AIDS substantially. However, the treatment 'roll-out' will take time, and given the government's ongoing concerns about 'affordability', it is unlikely to reach many (if not most) of those who need it.

The burden of AIDS will thus continue to be borne unevenly in South Africa. This is largely because of South Africa's high unemployment rate and the strong connection between unemployment, poverty and HIV-infection. Whereas the bulk of people living with AIDS cannot afford HAART, a small, but growing, number can access it through their companies or medical schemes. This enables them to live longer, more productive lives and cushions the impact of AIDS on economic growth. Until the public sector HAART programme can reach significant numbers of poor people living with AIDS, the income gulf between the employed and the unemployed will continue to harden into a socio-economic divide bringing life to one side and death to the other. The amount of resources allocated to combating AIDS (through prevention and treatment interventions) thus has major implications for the nature of South African society.

This study of the moral economy of AIDS policy in South Africa illustrates how economic analysis can help government and civil society think about addressing AIDS. Economics provides a powerful set of conceptual tools that enable us to decide how best to allocate scarce resources. But in the process, assumptions have to be made about social preferences and objectives. This normative aspect of economic analysis is often hidden or underplayed by the discourse of expertise employed by policy economists. This book uses economic tools to address the costs and benefits of various policy options, but it does so in an accessible manner and is at pains to highlight the implicit normative assumptions and implications. This is why the term 'moral economy' (rather than just 'economics') is used in the title. AIDS is far more than an economic problem. The way it is addressed cuts to the heart of what it means to be a society or what Rorty (1996) calls a 'moral community'.

The term 'moral economy' was first coined by E. P. Thompson in his discussion of the bread and food riots in eighteenth-century England. Such forms of popular dissent, he argued, were 'legitimised by an older moral economy, which taught the immorality of any unfair method of forcing up the price of provisions by profiteering upon the necessities of the people' (1963: 63). They comprised a 'last desperate effort by the people to reimpose the older moral economy as against the economy of the free market' (ibid. 67). Such protest was mirrored in other parts of Europe during the seventeenth and eighteenth centuries as capitalist forms of production transformed social and economic relationships.

James Scott, in his classic analysis of the 'moral economy of the peasant', argued that the deeply felt 'right to subsistence' characterised not only European working class struggles, but also peasant protest and resistance in South Asia, China, Latin America and Russia:

The operating assumption of the 'right to subsistence' is that all members of a community have a presumptive right to a living so far as local resources will allow. This subsistence claim is morally based on the common notion of a hierarchy of human needs, with the means for physical survival naturally taking priority over all other claims to village wealth. In a purely logical sense, it is difficult to imagine how any disparities in wealth and resources can be legitimated unless the right to subsistence is given priority. This right is surely the minimal claim that an individual makes on his society and is perhaps the reason that it has such moral force (1976: 176–7).

With the destruction of pre-industrial forms of subsistence and social relations, the state emerged in liberal democracies as a regulator of market relationships and a provider of poor relief/welfare for the indigent. As Polyani (1957) has shown, this reconstitution of the relationship between state, society and economy was essential for sustainable capitalist development. Citizens accepted market forces and economic inequality as legitimate – as long as the state guaranteed basic support for the unemployed, promoted full-employment policies, facilitated a degree of redistribution through the budget and regulated the working environment.

That the state had a duty to provide for the basic subsistence needs of the poor became an accepted principle of justice within liberal capitalist democracies (Rawls 1993). To the extent that a 'moral economy' of the welfare state can be discerned, it was one in which the welfare state guaranteed both political citizenship (through the universal franchise) and social citizenship (Marshall 1950), i.e. a minimum subsistence income and protection from the worst excesses of the market.

In South Africa, where high unemployment is linked to poverty and inequality, a broad-based coalition has emerged in favour of a universal basic income grant (BIG). South Africa's welfare system provides relatively generous support for the elderly, the young and the disabled. However, it is premised on full employment and thus provides limited (if any) social assistance to the unemployed (Nattrass and Seekings 1997). Given that over a third of the labour force is unemployed, this constitutes a very large hole in the welfare net. A BIG would help provide food security and can be located with the moral economy of a 'right to subsistence'. Can a similar case be made for implementing AIDS prevention and treatment intervention on a sufficiently massive scale that it reaches all who need it? Is there a deeply held presumption among South Africans that all people have a right to be protected from AIDS and given treatment when they become infected? Put differently, do people believe in the right to be protected from hunger *and* ill-health in the face of a major pandemic?

In addressing this question, it is important to distinguish between attitudes towards AIDS prevention, and attitudes towards AIDS treatment. There appears to be no discernible political constituency in South Africa which believes that AIDS should *not* be combated through prevention interventions (although people disagree over which strategies are most effective). Everyone seems to favour AIDS prevention interventions, and this book takes the need for AIDS prevention interventions as a given. The controversial issue relates primarily to treating AIDS – i.e. providing HAART for all people living with AIDS (see Chapter 4 for more details).

According to a recent national survey, 97% of South Africans believe that the government should use antiretrovirals to combat the spread of HIV from mother to child, and 95% believe that HAART should be given to those living with AIDS (Shisana and Simbayi 2002: 91). While this indicates strong support in principle for AIDS treatment, one cannot conclude that South Africans are necessarily in favour of prioritising treatment over other social objectives. This is because people's attitudes to spending vary dramatically once a trade-off is posed. For example, in a recent survey of working-class Cape Town, 60% of respondents 'agreed strongly' that the government should increase the old-age pension. However, when asked whether the old-age pension should be increased 'even if it means that people like you have to pay higher taxes' the proportion of respondents who agreed strongly fell by half to 27% and the proportion who disagreed strongly rose tenfold, from 3% to 29% (Seekings 2003c: 14–15).

The most we can conclude from the national survey is that *if* there are no resource constraints, the vast majority of South Africans would be in favour of AIDS treatment. This is a very different proposition to the moral economy conception of a 'right to subsistence' which has, across different societies and over the course of history, been seen as 'taking priority over all other claims' on social wealth. We have no idea how the respondents to the survey would have ranked AIDS treatment if they had been presented with a choice between a full-scale AIDS treatment programme or spending more resources on, say, crime prevention, or a BIG, or improved schooling.

Furthermore, the demand for the government to provide AIDS treatment to all who need it does not carry the same universal moral force as the 'right to subsistence'. As discussed in this book, there are strong moral, economic and public health arguments in favour of providing HAART to people living with AIDS. But these are not the only arguments which can be (and are) brought to bear on the subject. For example, it is possible to argue that the state does not have an obligation to provide treatment to those who, in the course of exercising free choice, ignore the available information about AIDS and contract the disease through unsafe sex. As Benatar has demonstrated, a consistent moral argument can be constructed to the effect that 'those who are responsible for their predicament are not morally entitled to such services' (2002: 394).[1] AIDS activists, of course, disagree – arguing that the right to life is paramount (e.g. Cameron 2001). In March 2003, the Treatment Action Campaign (TAC) charged the minister of health with culpable homicide for 'unlawfully and negligently' causing the death of people living with AIDS (by failing to provide HAART in the public sector) and thereby breaching her 'constitutional duty to respect, promote and fulfil the right to life and dignity of these people' (TAC 2003).

Not enough is known about the strength of public support for providing HAART to argue that this amounts to a deeply embedded moral belief about the duty of the state to provide it for all who need it as a basic right. However, it is possible to explore the *implicit* moral economy assumptions underpinning the government's AIDS policy. Despite high levels of public support (in principle) for HAART, successive ministers of health have argued that the use of antiretroviral medication to combat AIDS, either as a means of preventing unborn children from contracting the virus or to treat those already infected, was 'unaffordable'. This discourse shifted slightly in 2003 once it became clear that public pressure in favour of AIDS treatment was making a HAART intervention inevitable. Rather than arguing that HAART was simply unaffordable, government officials started stressing that the future treatment intervention had to be 'sustainable', i.e. within the limits set by available resources. While sustainability is obviously desirable, the term begs the obvious question of how many resources should be allocated to AIDS treatment.

By locating the AIDS policy discussion in a seemingly technical discourse of affordability and sustainability, the space for public deliberation over the appropriate size of a national treatment programme has been sharply curtailed. This has had the effect of stifling the formulation and expression of social values concerning how best to address the AIDS pandemic. It has also undermined any discussion of whether people are prepared to pay higher taxation in order to support a large-scale treatment intervention that reaches all who need it. Instead, the discourse of affordability and cost-effectiveness effectively insulates the AIDS policy debate from any discussion of raising the additional revenue through taxation.

A central objective of this book is to facilitate informed social debate about AIDS policy in South Africa. But it also has relevance beyond South Africa's borders and should be of interest to all those interested in the moral economy of AIDS policy in developing countries. The discourse of 'unaffordability' is not uniquely South African. Although there is a growing chorus of voices (activist, academic[2] and international[3]) in favour of AIDS treatment, there remains a conventional wisdom in economics that developing countries either cannot afford it at all, or can only afford a very limited treatment intervention.

According to Farmer *et al.*: 'There is an unmentioned elephant in the conference rooms of many scientific meetings: the prospect of providing HAART to those living with both poverty and HIV' (2001: 404). Economic cost-effectiveness studies have attempted to estimate the size of this 'unmentioned elephant' by showing that the marginal dollar spent on prevention delivers a better dividend in terms of HIV-infections averted than the marginal dollar spent on treatment (see e.g. Creese *et al.* 2002 and Marseille *et al.* 2002). As discussed later on, such studies do not grapple adequately with the link between AIDS treatment and prevention.

Providing HAART to people with AIDS helps prevent new infections for two reasons. Firstly, it lowers their viral load, thereby making them less infectious (e.g. Vernazza *et al.* 2002; UNAIDS 1999a; Quin *et al.* 2000). Secondly, if HAART is available, more people are likely to participate in voluntary counselling and testing, which in turn is likely to promote safer sexual behaviour (see Chapters 4 and 5). These two effects suggest that treating people with HAART not only prolongs their lives but saves the lives of others by preventing new HIV infections. According to the ASSA2000 Interventions Model, more than a million new HIV infections (over a 14 year period) could be prevented if a full-scale national treatment programme was implemented (see Chapter 4).

Conventional cost-effectiveness studies have a further weakness in that they are typically conducted within a narrow frame of reference. Cost components and output measures vary between studies, thus making comparison difficult (Freedberg and Yazdanpanah 2003). They also tend to focus mainly on the direct cost of HAART (e.g. drugs, personnel costs, etc.) without giving adequate consideration to the fact that the inter-vention may well save resources elsewhere in the health sector (Creese *et al.* 2002). A HAART programme is likely to lower AIDS-related morbidity among AIDS patients and result in fewer new HIV infections (and associ-ated subsequent morbidity). Fewer people will thus need hospitalisation for AIDS-related illness if a HAART programme was in place than would be the case if one was not. Indeed, Brazilian research indicates that such cost-savings to the health sector may well exceed the cost of the HAART programme (Texiera *et al.* 2003). Chapters 3 and 4 show that when the 'savings' associated with lower AIDS-related morbidity are factored into the cost-benefit analysis for South Africa, the 'net' costs of providing a full-scale AIDS intervention (including HAART) are significantly lower than implied by the direct costs.

By concentrating on the direct costs of interventions, cost-effectiveness studies typically reflect the perspective of a budget manager or a foreign aid donor – rather than that of the entire domestic health sector or the society in general. This book looks at the economics of AIDS through a much wider lens. It presents a view from the perspective of a middle-income African country considering the broader resource implications of responding to the AIDS pandemic. The analysis is not structured by the question 'should the marginal Rand[4] be allocated to prevention or treat-ment', but rather asks 'how much would it cost South Africa to reach all citizens through a large-scale package of AIDS prevention and treatment programmes'. Whereas the typical marginal analysis is a useful tool for technocratic decision makers working within the context of a limited budget, the analysis presented here allows questions to be asked about the appropriate size of the health budget. The normative and social dimensions of AIDS policy are discussed alongside the economic analysis.

This book takes the science of HIV and AIDS as given. For a useful summary of the evidence in this regard, see NIAID (2000).[5] It also accepts the large body of evidence indicating that antiretroviral medication is an effective means of facilitating mother-to-child transmission prevention (MTCTP) and extending the lives of people living with AIDS. According to a recent study of 9,803 HAART patients in seventy countries, the initial drop in mortality and morbidity after the introduction of HAART was sustained and potential long-term adverse effects associated with HAART did not alter its effectiveness in treating AIDS (Mocroft *et al.* 2003). This book accepts the findings of such empirical studies, i.e. it assumes that HAART is effective, and concentrates attention on the issue of whether HAART is 'unaffordable'.

1.1 An overview of the book

South Africa is a particularly interesting case study of the moral and economic challenges posed by a major AIDS pandemic. In 2003 an estimated 21.5% of South Africans aged 15–59 were HIV-positive, with over a thousand people dying each day of AIDS.[6] South Africa is a middle-income industrialised country with a relatively well-developed public health sector and (since 1994) a democratic political system. The prospects for a strong and effective response towards AIDS were thus, on the face of it, promising. Unfortunately the old apartheid regime failed to act effectively against the pandemic and, despite initial hopes, the new democratic government's response to AIDS was soon mired in controversy and inaction (see Chapter 2).

As can be seen in Table 1.1, South Africa has a per capita income similar to that of Brazil and Botswana. But unlike the governments of these countries, the South African government resisted calls to introduce an AIDS treatment programme until August 2003, when the cabinet finally agreed to consider it. The contrast with Brazil, where universal access to HAART has been a principle driving health policy since 1996 (Texiera *et al.* 2003), is particularly striking. However, on one level the comparison with Brazil is perhaps unfair. Brazil's AIDS pandemic is typical of the United States of America and other industrialised countries (Parker 2000) in that

Table 1.1 *South Africa in a comparative context*

	Brazil	Botswana	South Africa
Total population (2001)	172,559,000	1,554,000	43,792,000
Gross national per capita income (US$) (1999)	$4,350	$3,240	$3,170
% of government budget spent on health (1998)	9.0%	5.5%	11.6%
Life expectancy at birth (1995–2000)	67	44	57
Infant mortality rate per 1,000 live births (1995–2000)	42	74	58
HIV prevalence among adults	0.7%	38.8%	20.1%
Number of HIV-positive people	610,000	330,000	5,000,000
Deaths due to AIDS in 2001	8,400	26,000	360,000
AIDS treatment programmes	Free public provision of HAART from 1996.	Limited public provision of HAART (since 2002). Large companies also provide HAART to their workers.	Some private companies started providing HAART in 2001. In August 2003 the government agreed to provide HAART through the public health sector.

Source: UNAIDS, 2002 epidemiological fact sheets on Brazil, Botswana and South Africa. Available on www.unaids.org

it originated primarily among gay men and injecting drug-users (mainly in urban areas) and was able to be contained through early, targeted, interventions and free access to antiretrovirals (Texiera *et al.* 2003). South Africa's pandemic is typically African, i.e. it is characterised by hetero-sexual transmission and is strongly linked to poverty and transport links, with high HIV-prevalence areas in the region (see Section 1.2). It thus spread much faster and posed far greater challenges for AIDS prevention and treatment than the Brazilian pandemic. Nevertheless, the fact that Botswana, with substantially higher HIV prevalence than South Africa, took the bold step in 2002 of rolling out a treatment programme in key sites (Ramotlhwa 2003), indicates that the defining difference is probably related largely to political will. By the end of 2004 it is likely that various AIDS treatment sites will be available in the South African public health sector. But the scale of the treatment intervention in relation to the number of people who need it, is likely to be limited.

Unlike South Africa, Botswana has made a concerted attempt to obtain additional support from the Gates Foundation and the Global Fund for AIDS, Tuberculosis and Malaria to finance a treatment programme. Also unlike South Africa, Botswana (along with nineteen other countries who are using the United Nations Accelerated Access Initiative to obtain preferential pricing of HAART) has engaged in negotiations with pharmaceutical companies over the price of antiretrovirals (Lucchini *et al.* 2003: 175–6). Although the HAART programme in Botswana is reaching only a small proportion of people who need treatment (UNAIDS 2002b: 19–20) there is political commitment to the ongoing expansion of this programme (Ramotlhwa 2003).

Faced with government inertia in South Africa, TAC was formed by AIDS activists in December 1998 to campaign for affordable treatment for all people living with HIV/AIDS (TAC 2001). TAC has successfully put pressure on the government to improve AIDS policy, on drug companies to lower prices, and has promoted AIDS awareness and treatment literacy. In 2002 TAC won a constitutional court case forcing the government to implement a national MTCTP programme. The roll-out, however, was slow and uneven (see Chapter 3).

Having secured victory on MTCTP, TAC then turned its attention to the issue of providing HAART for those who are ill with AIDS. A process of discussion and negotiation between representatives of labour, government and civil society (notably TAC) was conducted under the auspices of South Africa's peak-level tripartite institution, the National Economic Development and Labour Council (NEDLAC). This process appeared to have resulted in an 'agreement' at the end of 2002, but the government subsequently muddied the waters by refusing to sign it. In 2003 TAC embarked on a civil disobedience campaign over the issue, but called it off in April after the government reopened discussions on AIDS treatment. In response to continued government procrastination, TAC restarted its civil disobedience campaign in August and announced that it was considering legal action against the government. A week later the cabinet pronounced in favour of AIDS treatment, and gave the health minister until the end of September to produce a 'detailed operational plan'.

These policy victories, while important, are limited and constrained by a government that controls the scale, pace and nature of implementation. Continued distrust of antiretroviral interventions (be they for MTCTP or HAART) by high-level officials, coupled with the ongoing hegemonic discourse of 'unaffordability', means that South Africa is still a long way from providing the kind of comprehensive AIDS interventions found in Brazil.

Chapter 2 provides an overview of the development of AIDS policy in South Africa. It describes the implicit moral economy of current AIDS policy as a 'moral economy of triage' whereby the majority of those with AIDS are denied HAART on the grounds that it is 'unaffordable'. Chapters 3 and 4 question the economic and normative logic of this policy stance. Chapter 3 argues that far from being 'unaffordable', an MTCTP programme will almost certainly save the government money. Chapter 4 outlines the costs and benefits (in terms of fewer new HIV infections, fewer orphans, etc.) of a large-scale AIDS intervention including HAART. It shows that the social benefits of including HAART as part of a broader AIDS intervention are substantial, and that the economic costs are within the bounds of the feasible.

The demographic model used in Chapter 4 assumes that a HAART intervention has strong preventive characteristics. As discussed earlier, this is because of the impact of voluntary counselling and testing on behaviour, and the effect of HAART on viral loads. However, as the relationship between HAART and behaviour change is controversial (with some people worrying that HAART could result in an increase in risky sex), Chapter 5 considers this issue in more detail. It is argued that the balance of evidence indicates that including HAART in an AIDS intervention programme will help prevent new HIV infections.

Chapter 4 examines the economics of providing HAART from a health budget perspective. But there are other economic benefits that should also be considered – such as the impact on companies and households. The provision of HAART (or failure to provide it) has implications that extend to productivity growth, structural change, and inequality. Chapter 6 considers the impact of AIDS on economic growth, and draws implications from firm-level studies of business responses. The chapter reviews the existing macroeconomic models of the impact of AIDS in South Africa. All show that AIDS will lower growth, but two out of the three major models predict that population growth will slow down faster than aggregate output – thus bringing about an increase in per capita income. This raises the possibility that AIDS may reduce the size of the economic pie, but that each remaining person will get a larger slice. It is not impossible that

Malthusian projections such as these may have contributed to the government's reluctance to act more decisively against AIDS. However, as Chapter 6 explains, the output of macroeconomic modelling is profoundly affected by theoretical and empirical assumptions. Caution must thus be exercised when considering their predictions.

Given the lack of adequate welfare support for the unemployed, and the strong connection between unemployment and poverty, we are confronted with the need to address AIDS and poverty. Chapter 7 concludes the book by arguing that there are strong grounds for introducing both a BIG and a large-scale AIDS prevention and treatment intervention.

Why focus on AIDS?

What is it about AIDS that singles out the disease for special attention over other life-threatening diseases such as malaria or tuberculosis (TB)? One answer is to point to the link between HIV and these other diseases. The AIDS pandemic is probably contributing to the spread of malaria and TB in Africa (Corbett *et al.* 2002; Godfrey-Faussett *et al.* 2002) and hence trying to fight malaria and TB instead of AIDS does not necessarily make sense. Another answer to the question is that AIDS is different because it constitutes a public health crisis and a threat to economic livelihood akin to no other illness. As De Cock *et al.* put it:

HIV / AIDS is the greatest threat to life, liberty and the pursuit of happiness and prosperity in many African countries. Interventions, therefore, must be quantitatively and qualitatively commensurate with the magnitude of the threat posed by the disease (2002: 68).

De Waal makes a similar point, arguing that the impact of AIDS on economic development amounts to a 'development process run in reverse' (2003: 11).

AIDS is diabolical in that it affects mainly prime-age adults and has a long incubation period between stage 1 (no symptoms) and stage 4 (full-blown AIDS). Unless people get tested, they can be passing on the virus through sexual intercourse without knowing it. This makes the disease very hard to contain. Furthermore, by harnessing the basic human desire for sexual intimacy (and the breastfeeding of babies) as the prime means of transmission, the virus can gain a fast and extensive grip on an entire population, leaving heartbreak and socio-economic devastation in its wake. And, as economic hardship increases, so too does the risk of HIV transmission. These biological and socio-economic aspects of AIDS make the disease a worthy target for special policy attention.

Section 1.2 discusses the socio-economic determinants of AIDS, focussing specifically on the two horns of the development dilemma: the positive relationship between poverty and AIDS; and the negative relationship between AIDS and economic growth. Section 1.3 then poses the question of how to respond. The discussion here is primarily philosophical. It outlines a central tenet of the book, namely that technical economic analysis can be a useful tool for social decision-making, but only if it enhances understanding and informs debate.

1.2 The socio-economic determinants of AIDS in Africa

HIV/AIDS is having a devastating impact on development in Africa.[7] According to the World Bank, if the AIDS pandemic had not happened in Southern Africa, 'life expectancy would have reached 64 by 2010–15. Instead, it will have regressed to 47, reversing the gains of the past 30 years' (2001: 139). Figure 1.1 shows how life expectancy rose in the ten Southern African countries during the 1970s and early 1980s, but then fell sharply in the 1990s as the AIDS pandemic and economic crisis took their toll.

About half the total number of HIV-positive Southern Africans live in South Africa, where death rates have increased dramatically in the age group 15–39. The AIDS pandemic is clearly implicated in this increase. As Dr Makgoba, the former head of South Africa's Medical Research Council, pointed out, only a war could result in comparable deaths among young people (cited in Van der Vliet 2000).

But unlike a war situation, the increase in mortality has been borne disproportionately by women (especially young women). Figure 1.2 shows a sharp increase in the number of deaths of South African women in their twenties over the past five years. This is a function of the biology of HIV infection (women are more easily infected than men[8]), and of the social and economic disadvantages experienced by women (Walker and Gilbert 2002; IFAD 2001: 9–11). This pattern of increased vulnerability of women to HIV infection is replicated across Africa (see UNAIDS 1999 and Baylies and Bujra 2001: 1–24).

Poverty and AIDS

From the mid-1970s to the end of the century, the AIDS pandemic claimed 14 million lives, which, as Cooper points out, is a 'holocaust equal in magnitude (but over fewer years) to the slave trade' (2002: 110). Why is it that AIDS has proved so much more deadly in Africa than anywhere else in the world? Part of the answer may have to do with the type of HIV

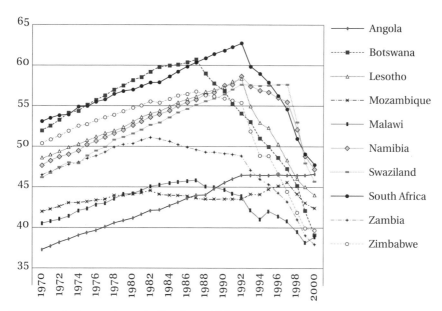

Figure 1.1 *Life expectancy in Southern Africa*
Source: World Bank data from WEFA

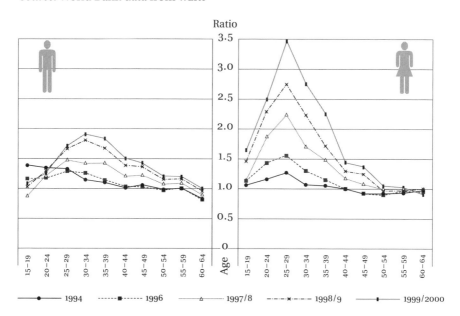

Figure 1.2 *Increase in adult death rates in South Africa*
Source: Dorrington *et al.* 2001: 29

virus found in Africa. Although there is no conclusive evidence, some researchers suspect that HIV-1C, which appears to have a higher replicative rate and concentration in bodily fluids, may be more infectious than the HIV-1B virus found in the United States and Europe (Cherry 2002). But the roots of African susceptibility go deeper than this and include its history of colonialism and slavery; sustained civil and military conflict; geographic disadvantage; patterns of migration; poor governance and structural adjustment (Barnett and Whiteside 2002: 124–56). South Africa, with its transport[9] and labour links into Southern Africa, was unfortunately well placed to experience a rapidly moving AIDS pandemic. As Decosas describes, there is a

[c]rescent-shaped distribution of high HIV prevalence extending from Namibia in the south-west along the east coast to Kenya, then via Southern Sudan into the Central African Republic. As in the West African region, the southern horn of this crescent coincides with a zone of intense labour migration to a single destination, South Africa (1998: 167).

South Africa's history of participating in military struggles in the region (by the old apartheid army and the liberation forces) may also have contributed to the spread of AIDS. Shell writes:

As early as 1976, South African apartheid soldiers invaded Angola and other neighbouring HIV-infected countries. After apartheid collapsed, approximately 40,000 returning cadres from all liberation groups who were living in those same frontline countries, and some deeper in HIV-devastated Africa, were incorporated into the new SANDF (South African National Defence Force) without a single HIV-test. After induction, they were distributed to all military installations throughout the country, i.e. in a systematic pattern across the landscape. If one were to design a pandemic, this would be the perfect blueprint (1999: 147–8).

Early analytical approaches to the global AIDS pandemic focussed on the pathogen (the HI virus) and on the individual behavioural determinants of HIV transmission. This focussed attention on high-risk groups (e.g. migrant workers, truck drivers, soldiers and commercial sex workers) as 'vectors' of the spread of HIV. Subsequent analysis shifted attention more towards sexual culture and high-risk behaviours (as opposed to high-risk groups). In East Africa, risky sexual cultural practices include widow inheritance, widow 'cleansing', wife sharing, wife exchanging with land and cattle, polygamy and female circumcision (United Nations 2003). In Southern Africa, socio-cultural norms of gender inequality, sexual violence, a preference for dry sex,[10] fatalistic attitudes and pressures to prove fertility contribute to a high-risk environment (Leclerc-Madlala 2001, 2002; Eaton *et al.* 2003; Wojcicki and Malala 2001; Wojcicki 2002).

Sexual culture is an important dimension of the AIDS pandemic (Crothers 2001; Alexander and Uys 2002) and is discussed in more detail in Chapter 5. Understanding it contributes to our knowledge of HIV transmission (especially the vulnerability of young women) and of the challenges faced by interventions designed to change behaviour. Recently, the National AIDS Councils/Commissions of Kenya, Uganda and Tanzania issued a statement recognising the 'centrality of culture' to the AIDS pandemic and urging the need to 'transform' it (United Nations 2003). However, this can be a difficult task, particularly when it comes to transforming sexual relationships in a context where men are expected to have multiple sexual partnerships, and where young women form sexual liaisons with older men for financial advantage. As the following report from Tanzania suggests, older men and young women are locked in a sexual culture which exposes them all to HIV infection:

A commonly heard saying about AIDS goes accordingly: *Acha Iniue, Dogo-dogo Sintaacha* [in Swahili, 'let it kill me but I will not leave the young girls']. Although this statement is sometimes said by bragging men, it is not merely men's talk or wishful expression of their maleness, but is rather expressing a social reality in male-female sexual relations (Haram 2001: 50).

This 'social reality' is one in which the power relations are skewed in favour of men, and where sex is a currency by which African women and girls are frequently 'expected to pay for life's opportunities, from a passing grade in school to a trading license or permission to cross a border' (UNAIDS quoted in Baylies and Bujra 2001: 7). The trading of sexual favours out of desperation has been dubbed 'survival sex' (Wojcicki 2002: 268). A report from Zambia during the recent famine revealed that women were charging two Zambian dollars for sex – and double if the man did not want to use a condom. According to the local medical officer, these women were 'educated about the virus, but say that they would rather die of AIDS than hunger' (*Mail and Guardian,* 1–7 November 2002).

However, women do not always participate in the sexual economy simply out of desperation (Wojcicki and Malala 2001; Hunter 2002). According to Leclerc-Madlala, there is evidence that for some young Zulu women sexuality is conceptualised as a resource that can be drawn upon for material or economic advantage. For example, sex can be used to secure a job or to acquire material benefits of various kinds from men. The sexual economy operates on a continuum or 'scale of benefits'. This ranges from the trading by women of sexual favours in order to secure basic needs (i.e. food, school fees and rents) to the use of sex for obtaining expensive fashion accessories (e.g. clothes), prestigious outings (e.g. invitations to dine at restaurants and attend cinemas) and the opportunity to ride in luxury cars or sleep in hotels (2002: 31).

Men, in turn, are expected to provide money and gifts in return for sex. As the Nigerian saying goes, 'there is no romance without finance' (cited in Barnett and Whiteside 2002: 85).

Unfortunately, the price for participating in this 'sexual economy' is greater vulnerability to HIV infection, especially for young women. LeBeau *et al.* observe that when Namibian men expect to get sex as 'change' (i.e. in exchange) for the money they spend on women, it becomes harder for women to request safe sex because money is involved (2001: 63–5). Kelly and Ntlabati draw similar conclusions from South African research, pointing out that when relationships are premised on money and the need for status, these are 'circumstances in which young women have little power to insist on condom use' (2002: 52).

But sexual culture cannot alone (or even significantly) explain the virulence of the spread of AIDS in Africa. According to a study of the determinants of HIV infection in four sub-Saharan African cities, high rates of partner change, contacts with commercial sex workers, and concurrent sexual partnerships were not reported more systematically in the high-prevalence than in the low-prevalence sites (UNAIDS 1999b). Co-factors such as male circumcision (which appears to provide a degree of protection from HIV infection[11]), the presence of untreated sexually transmitted diseases (STDs) and the age of marriage for young women were highlighted by the study. Sexual behaviour is obviously an important driver of the pandemic – especially in Africa, where transmission is overwhelmingly heterosexual. But it is the *combination* of socio-economic and biomedical factors with unsafe sexual practices that produces the lethal basis for the spread of HIV.

More recent research has focussed on the immune system's response to HIV as a key determinant of HIV transmission. There is now a strong body of biomedical evidence showing that 'malnutrition and parasite infection increase HIV susceptibility, not only to opportunistic infection after HIV infection, but also to HIV transmission, just as they increase susceptibility to other infectious diseases' (Stillwaggon 2002: 4). Given that malnutrition is a function of poverty, there is thus good reason for assuming that poverty helped hasten the spread of HIV in sub-Saharan Africa. As Still-waggon observes, 'From 1988 to 1998, when nascent or concentrated AIDS epidemics developed into generalised epidemics in sub-Saharan Africa, 30% of the region was malnourished' (2002: 5). Micronutrient deficiencies (particularly of Vitamins A, C, and B) undermine the body's natural defences against HIV infection – i.e. skin integrity and mucous membranes – thus contributing further to the vulnerability to HIV infection. Parasite infections, mainly malaria, schistosomiasis (bilharzia), trypanosomiasis (sleeping sickness) and intestinal parasites undermine nutritional status and compromise the immune system yet further, effectively exhausting it. Such parasite infections are endemic in Africa, but the situation is made worse by inadequate health care – itself a function of poverty and low levels of development – which leaves most parasite infections untreated. Figure 1.3 summarises the links between poverty and HIV transmission.

Weak policy responses by most African governments no doubt also contributed to the AIDS pandemic. Poverty made the pandemic harder to fight, but it does not absolve the governments of responsibility for not acting faster and more aggressively against it. This is especially the case for South Africa which, as noted above, had more resources than other African countries to combat the AIDS pandemic. Most African governments themselves are now weakened by AIDS as the disease lowers productivity and efficiency, undermines the capacity to deliver services, and possibly even threatens democracy itself (Barnett and Whiteside 2002: 295–315; De Waal 2003).

As indicated in Figure 1.3, economic factors reinforce unsafe practices. Sexual culture places women in a vulnerable situation regarding HIV-infection, and poverty exacerbates it by encouraging women to engage in sex as an economic strategy for survival (Akeroyd 1997). Evidence from the demographic and health surveys in Southern Africa also indicates a strong connection between poverty and vulnerability to HIV-infection. According to Booysen's analysis of the data, poorer women know less about how HIV is transmitted, and are less able to access and use condoms, than their better-off counterparts (2002a: 403–4).

Education and skill also appear to influence vulnerability to HIV infec-tion. According to a national survey of South African youth, there were lower reported levels of sexual activity among better educated youth –

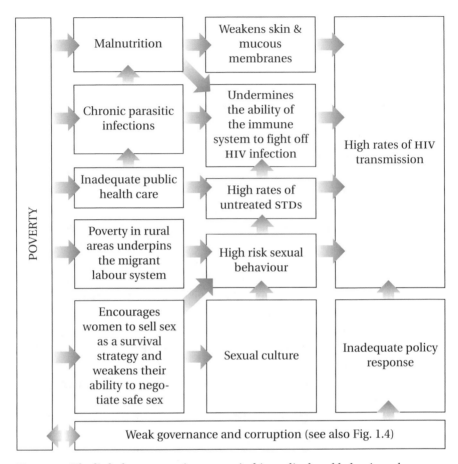

Figure 1.3 *The links between socio-economic, biomedical and behavioural determinants of the spread of AIDS in Africa*

particularly those living in urban areas (LoveLife 2000).[12] A national household survey found that those with tertiary educational qualifications had lower rates of HIV infection than those with only school-level qualifications (Shisana and Simbayi 2002: 54). Data from South African insurance companies indicate that those in the high skill bands have relatively low levels of HIV-infection (Dorrington 2001). A 2003 firm-based survey in Swaziland revealed a similar pattern (Evian 2003). As can be seen in Table 1.2, HIV prevalence falls sharply as skill level (and thus also the wage) rises. This trend is of greater significance than the impact of age on HIV prevalence.[13] The study concludes that younger workers are more vulnerable to

HIV infection, but that the higher vulnerability to HIV infection among lower-income/unskilled workers suggests that more attention should be paid to this group (Evian 2003: 13).

Table 1.2 *HIV prevalence in a large firm in Swaziland*

	Number tested (response rate)	% HIV-positive	95% confidence intervals
Job band			
1–3 (unskilled)	2,202 (58%)	42.6%	40.5%–44.7%
4–6 (semi-skilled)	772 (43%)	32.4%	29.2%–35.7%
7–11 (skilled)	454 (68%)	28.9%	24.8%–33.1%
12+ (highest skilled and professional)	179 (72%)	13.4%	9%–19%
Total permanent employment	3,607 (55%)	37.2%	35.7%–38.8%
Contract	268	35.1%	29.5%–40.9%
Seasonal	308	42.9%	37.4%–48.4%
Age band			
20–29	1,241	39.5%	36.8%–42.3%
30–39	1,151	41.5%	38.7%–44.4%
40–49	842	31.9%	28.9%–35.2%
50+	373	28.4%	24.0%–33.2%

Source: Evian (2003: 7, 8).

Findings such as these highlight education and economic development as important components of an integrated approach to combating AIDS. Providing more people with skills and access to better-paying jobs will probably pay off in terms of fewer HIV infections – although the announcement by the Anglo American corporation that HIV infection had reached the ranks of its senior managers,[14] indicates the limits of this kind of strategy. Education and skills development cannot be a substitute for serious policies to combat AIDS.

Ideally, structural issues such as the migrant labour system should also be addressed. Studies have shown that male migration from rural areas in search of employment (either on mines or in urban manufacturing) has contributed to high-risk environments in urban and rural areas. Migrant men living in hostels, and women living in the immediate vicinity of hostels, are particularly vulnerable to HIV infection (Williams *et al.* 2000). Women who remain behind in the rural areas have extramarital affairs, often selecting other migrant men, soldiers or taxi drivers (Dladla *et al.* 2001: 80). Migrant men involved in dangerous work on the mines appear to have adopted fatalistic attitudes towards HIV, which are particularly problematic in a high-risk environment for HIV infection (Campbell 1998; Macheke and Campbell 1998).

Does this link between economic factors and sexual behaviour mean that boosting growth and promoting economic development should be the main focus of a strategy to combat AIDS? Not necessarily. The second horn of the development dilemma – i.e. the fact that AIDS undermines growth and development – makes the policy challenge much more complex than simply prioritising poverty alleviation. Ultimately, an effective strategy against AIDS requires a combination of anti-AIDS interventions and pro-poor development strategies.

AIDS and economic growth

AIDS undermines economic security and growth in various ways. It reduces the economic security of households by reducing the productivity of (and eventually killing) income-earners, while simultaneously diverting scarce household resources towards medical expenditure. This double squeeze on household security is increasingly well documented in the growing body of research on the impact of AIDS on households in South and Southern Africa.[15] Women are especially hard-hit because they carry the burden of the disease and yet are expected to care for other members of the household who are also HIV positive (Walker and Gilbert 2002: 82).[16]

There is a growing body of South African research showing that AIDS can be devastating at household level (e.g. Desmond *et al.* 2000; Steinberg *et al.* 2002a, 2002b; Booysen *et al.* 2002). In most of sub-Saharan Africa, where agriculture accounts for a significant portion of employment and output, HIV/AIDS is having an especially detrimental impact on rural households engaged in peasant agriculture (IFAD 2001; De Waal and Tumushabe 2003):

The epidemic has caused the decimation of skilled and unskilled agricultural labour; a steep reduction in smallholder agricultural production; a decline in commercial agriculture; the loss of indigenous farming methods, inter-generational knowledge and specialised skills and practices; and capacity erosion and disruption in the service delivery of formal and informal rural institutions resulting from the scale of staff morbidity and mortality. (IFAD 2001: iv)

AIDS in sub-Saharan Africa thus threatens food security directly through its impact on peasant agriculture. By contrast, South Africa's experience of de-agrarianisation and the destruction of peasant agriculture under apartheid, resulted in a situation where most food is produced by large, capital-intensive commercial farms. According to the February 2002 Labour Force Survey, only 7% of employment in South Africa was in subsistence and small-scale agriculture. Given that only a small proportion of household income is generated by subsistence agriculture, the bulk of this 'employment' is in fact large-scale underemployment. The impact of AIDS on the economic security of poor households in South Africa is thus felt primarily through declining income rather than food production. The impact of AIDS at firm-level is thus of particular importance in South Africa (see Chapter 6).

AIDS reduces productivity at work and increases production costs for firms (Avetin and Huard 2000; McPherson *et al.* 2000; Fox *et al.* 2003). This, together with the negative impact of AIDS on income and consumption, slows growth. Government efficiency is also likely to be undermined by AIDS – thus reducing the capacity of the government to deliver social and economic services (De Waal 2003). Slower growth in turn reduces the tax capacity of the economy, thus undermining the potential developmental role for the state. Household economic security is thus threatened *directly* (through the morbidity and mortality of household members) and *indirectly* (via the negative 'second-round' impact of AIDS on the broader economy and on the government). Rising levels of poverty in turn increase vulnerability to HIV infection, which in turn lowers growth, thus generating more poverty and vulnerability to HIV. This is a vicious spiral indeed. These connections are summarised in Figure 1.4.

The impact of AIDS on economic growth in South Africa is discussed in more detail in Chapter 6. The purpose of this brief discussion is simply to highlight the various economic pathways by which AIDS impacts negatively on growth. The dynamics summarised in Figures 1.3 and 1.4 highlight the development dilemma posed by AIDS for low- and middle-income developing countries.

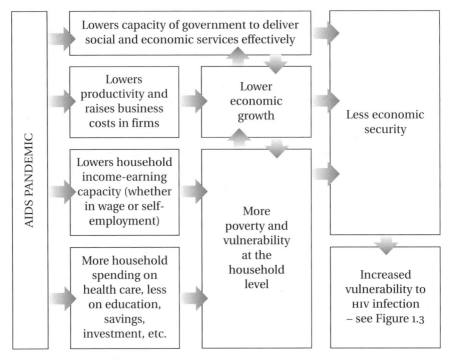

Figure 1.4 AIDS *and economic security*

1.3 Economic analysis and the development dilemma

The link between poverty and AIDS in Africa poses a development dilemma[17] which can be summarised as follows:

1 Poverty contributes to the spread of AIDS (Fig. 1.3).

2 AIDS treatment and prevention programmes are more effective when people are well nourished.

Therefore: *poverty alleviation is a precondition for combating* AIDS. But:

3 AIDS undermines productivity and economic growth (Fig. 1.4).

4 Economic growth is necessary for sustainable poverty alleviation.

Therefore: *addressing* AIDS *is a precondition for addressing poverty.*

What, then, is the appropriate way forward? Is there an 'optimal' set of policies which balance the need to address AIDS now (in order to ensure growth later) with the need to support growth (so as to lower HIV-infection rates later)? Reflecting on this problem, Poku observes that Africa's challenge is to achieve 'the sustainable development essential for an effective response to the pandemic under conditions where the pandemic is destructive of the capacities essential for the response – namely, killing the most economically productive members of the continent's people'. He concludes that 'simple answers to this problem do not exist, but recognition of its nature is a step towards its solution' (2002: 545).

But is this really the nature of the problem? Is the development challenge simply one of what economists call 'constrained optimisation', i.e. maximising growth given the constraints imposed by AIDS on human resources (i.e. the fact that it is killing off prime-age adults)? If the problem is conceptualised *solely* as one of constrained development, then one possible 'rational' response might be to concentrate on protecting the most productive individuals (because they contribute most to growth) and otherwise devote resources to enhancing growth. Such a strategy may include giving HIV-negative people preferential access to welfare, education and health services and even confining HIV-positive people to 'sanitoria' (as in Cuba[18]) or the equivalent of leper colonies.

The problem with this line of logic is obvious: if you concentrate resources on the 'most productive members of society' in order to maximise growth, you sacrifice the ideal of equal treatment and respect for persons. It conjures up a vision of a brutal (and brutalising) society in which the HIV-positive are shunned and discriminated against in an effort to ensure a greater share of income for those who survive the pandemic. Society, in short, could be fundamentally reshaped by such a technocratic 'no compassion' approach. Not surprisingly, then, democratic governments (even in poor countries) baulk at it. The approach may be 'rational' on one level, but many of the policy recommendations are 'unreasonable' in the sense that they are unlikely to be publicly endorsed in a democratic society of reasonable citizens.

Some philosophical underpinnings

The distinction between 'rational' and 'reasonable' is important and worthy of some consideration. Following Rawls, 'rational' agents use the powers of judgement and deliberation to seek their own ends, whereas 'reasonable' agents are 'ready to propose principles and standards as fair terms of co-operation and to abide by them willingly, given the assurance that others will likewise do so' (1993: 49–50).[19] The reasonable and the rational are complementary in a democratic society: 'Merely reasonable agents would have no ends of their own they wanted to advance by fair cooperation; merely rational agents lack a sense of justice and fail to recognise the independent validity of the claims of others' (1993: 52).[20] The importance of the reasonable is that it 'is public in a way that the rational is not' (ibid. 53). As Rawls argues, it is 'by the reasonable that we enter as equals the public world of others and stand ready to propose, or to accept, as the case may be, fair terms of co-operation with them ... Insofar as we are reasonable, we are ready to work out the framework for the public social world' (ibid.).

Economics is based on the assumption of rational decision making by individuals. Economic agents (be they citizens, companies or governments) use economic logic to achieve the best outcome for their objectives given a set of constraints. Reasonable discussion about social values has no direct place in economic analysis. As Paltiel observes, economics 'is an efficiency-driven science with no moral compass with regard to equity and compassion' (2000: 240–1). Rather, social norms enter standard economic analysis as 'exogenous' variables (i.e. determined outside the model) and are treated as 'constraints'. In the case of the possible policy responses to AIDS noted above, if reasonable people decide that it is unjust to provide unequal access to education and training to HIV-positive people, then the economist would take this 'constraint' into account and proceed accordingly. In terms of this intellectual framework, the role of the economist is simply to do the best *technical* job of allocating resources efficiently *given social preferences.*

But for social preferences to be manifest, public discussion is necessary. Economic analysis becomes dangerous when decision making power is ceded to seemingly technical arguments without realising the nature of the implicit social judgements behind them. This can happen when economists use what McCloskey (1990) calls the 'rhetoric of economic expertise' to intimidate critical voices and silence debate. For example, a minister of finance could invoke such rhetoric to defend a government's limited allocation of resources for HAART by saying that any increased expenditure would 'threaten to undermine the country's sound economic fundamentals'. As most people do not understand what this means (let alone that it is a contestable proposition), this use of the rhetoric of economic expertise effectively silences debate. Yet spending decisions by the government are also determined by political objectives (that are not always clear) and a host of debatable judgements about social preferences and economic behaviour. The economic 'experts' who work for and advise the government make all sorts of assumptions when informing decisions about how to allocate existing revenues (e.g. between armaments and AIDS treatment) and about the level of taxation they think that society is prepared to accept. These assumptions are disguised by their seemingly technical economic discourse.

When economists or policy makers make statements like 'it is not affordable to provide HAART to all those who need it', the use of the gnomic present – 'is not affordable' – conveys to the audience a sense of timeless truth. McCloskey argues that this discursive sleight of hand is typical of the rhetoric of economic expertise:

> The experts claim that their stories are 'positive, not normative', 'is' instead of 'ought', the way things are as against how they should be. The claim is at the centre of modernism. But stories carry an ethical burden. Concealing the ethical burden under a cloak of science is the master move of expertise (1990: 35).

Precisely such an 'ethical burden' lurks behind the claims made by South African government officials that providing MTCTP and HAART is 'unaffordable' or not 'cost-effective'. These terms are more than technical labels, as economic technocrats would have us believe. They are derived from a prior, and highly contestable, process of choice and analysis.

Public discussion is necessary to lay bare these social preferences and, more importantly, to shape and reshape them. This is why implicit in the notion of the 'reasonable' is its public nature. It is a central element of the idea of society (Rawls 1993: 49). Following Scanlon (1982), public discussion reflects the basic human desire to be able to justify our actions to others on grounds they could not reasonably reject. It is through public deliberation that social preferences are formulated and clarified. Without it, society is impoverished, and decision-making space is ceded to technocrats (including, importantly, economists). The danger posed by technocratic decision making is that value judgements are made by technocrats on behalf of society – and then disguised by the rhetoric of expertise. People are thus unaware that value judgements are being made on their behalf and are denied the opportunity to reflect on what values should inform public decision making about AIDS policy.

So far I have argued in favour of public discussion as a means of expressing and formulating the social values (the reasonable) that need to inform and guide the (rational) technocratic decision making about social allocation of resources. However, this rather idealistic depiction of the relationship between society and institutions of government fails to take into account the fact that institutions are not only shaped by social preferences, but in turn serve to shape social preferences. As Rothstein argues:

When one creates an institution by political means – for example, a social-insurance program, a tax system or a parliamentary forum for decision-making – one changes not only what future actors will regard as rational action. One changes *what they will regard as morally correct action as well.* The morality prevailing in society is, in other words, a product of the institutions built by that society's citizens and their representatives (1998: 138–9; emphasis in the original).

This bi-causal link between institutions and social norms poses something of a dilemma: what if the prevailing social norms are unjust? For example, in the case of slavery, prevailing social norms were both generated by and served to bolster the institution of slavery. Appealing to social norms thus does not necessarily guarantee a just outcome. Furthermore, people's interpretation of social norms and the construction of their own values and preferences are profoundly shaped by self-interest. Social institutions that facilitate co-ordinated and co-operative solutions to distributional conflict are built on the assumption of self-interested pursuit of objectives. Thus, for example, in the case of South Africa's tripartite institution, NEDLAC, organised labour negotiates in favour of policies that are in the interests of employed workers, and peak-level business organisations push for policies that support profitability. This kind of constituency-based behaviour is to be expected – and indeed is central to the very logic of such peak-level bargaining institutions. However, a corollary of this is that there is no guarantee that the resulting bargain will be beneficial to the wider-society.

In his classic work, Rawls (1971) addressed the problem of self-interested negotiation by means of a thought experiment. He models an 'original position' in which reasonable people come together to discuss the kind of society they would like to live in – but without knowing what social position they will hold, or the comprehensive doctrines they will live by. This 'veil of ignorance' effectively places the 'reasonable' pursuit of principles of justice prior to the 'rational' pursuit of individual self-interest. It models a pure public discursive process in which, he argues, reasonable people will select a social blueprint characterised by tolerance, respect for persons, and a conception of justice based on fairness.

Of course participants in real-world social discussions are products of their social context, have specific interests and competing notions of the social good. Does this mean that reasonable public discussion (i.e. divorced from matters of narrow self-interest) is impossible? Not necessarily. If we accept that people are motivated by self-interest *and* a basic human desire to be able to justify their actions to others on grounds they could not reasonably reject, then public discussion has a critical and emancipatory dimension. Yes, we are shaped by prevailing social norms, by our institutional and class context, and by our internally processed moral codes. But we can – at least to some extent – transcend these through critical self-reflection, and more importantly, through public discussion about what is just and how we should, as a society, conduct ourselves.

Habermas distinguishes between the 'formation and extension of critical theorems which can stand up to scientific discourse', social reflection on these theorems (in order to develop 'authentic insights'), and the selection of appropriate strategies to facilitate change (1974: 32). The events which led the shift in South African government policy on MTCTP (and subsequently on HAART) are examples of the interplay between these different processes. There was a scientific/economic challenge to the notion that the intervention was unaffordable (see Chapters 3 and 4); there was public debate and mobilisation on the issue; and finally there was the strategic decision on the part of AIDS activists to engage in legal challenges and civil disobedience. The MTCTP victory, however, was relatively easy as no one challenged the objective (to save the lives of children and save mothers the pain of having to pass on a terminal illness to their babies), and the resource implications were minor. The real challenge to society is the one confronting South Africa today: how to deal with poverty *and* implement a large-scale AIDS prevention and treatment intervention. As the resource implications are large, and the costs and benefits unevenly distributed across society, this social challenge is serious indeed.

When Habermas argues for social reflection and discourse as a means of shifting from 'true statements' to 'authentic insights', he is making two points, one practical and one theoretical. The practical point is a democratic one: that decisions about how to organise (or reorganise) society must ultimately lie with the public, i.e. technocratic information must be subject to public reflection. His theoretical point is that 'true statements' are meaningful only when they have been accepted by the public through a process of enlightened reflection. In making this argument, Habermas models the relationship between the social scientist and society as a therapeutic relationship akin to that between a psychological therapist and a patient.

This metaphor, however, does not fully capture the relationship between economic analysis and social reflection, discussion and negotiation. This is because so many assumptions about social values enter into economic analysis that it is often difficult (if not impossible) to separate scientific discourse from social reflection. The therapeutic relationship between social scientist and society runs in both directions. Economists can try to offer 'true statements' about trade-offs (true in the sense of logical and rational, given a set of clear assumptions), but economic analysis reflects 'authentic insights' only when social preferences are included in the decision model. This means that economists have to take society seriously in two ways: economic analysis must be clear about the assumptions that are being made about social preferences; and must be conducted in a way that encourages social reflection. The task is two-fold: to lay bare the choices and decisions about policies already being taken on behalf of the public; and to provide the best and most comprehensive analysis of the costs and benefits of alternative policy choices.

Paltiel and Stinnett refer to this as a 'prescriptive' or 'suggestive' economic approach, which seeks

to provide decision makers with information that can help them to make better choices but stops short of telling them what to do ... The goal of the approach is merely to structure choices to force decision makers to acknowledge their subjective assessments of value and to confront their implications (1998: 147–8).

In other words, economists can hold a mirror up to society and say 'this is the choice that your government is making. Do you like it?' The analysis provided in Chapter 2 of South African AIDS policy as a 'moral economy of triage' is an example of such an exercise.

2 AIDS policy in South Africa

South Africa is infamous for its obfuscation and prevarication on AIDS policy. It took a Constitutional Court ruling in 2002 to force the government to implement a national MTCTP intervention (and progress has subsequently been slow and uneven). Public pressure, a campaign of civil disobedience, and concerns about the 2004 election resulted, finally, in August 2003, in the government accepting the need for an AIDS treatment programme. Having accepted that antiretrovirals are beneficial, the major constraint on the roll-out of MTCTP and HAART is now the availability of resources. Given the ongoing discourse of affordability, it is argued that an implicit moral economy of triage informs the South African government's policy on AIDS.

2.1 A history of AIDS policy making in South Africa

The history of AIDS policy in South Africa is a sorry tale of missed opportunities, inadequate analysis, bureaucratic failure and political mismanagement. In the early 1990s, when the antenatal survey indicated that less than 3% of pregnant women attending government clinics were HIV-positive,[1] there were already clear warnings of an impending AIDS pandemic. Metropolitan Life's demographic model (the 'Doyle model') had established the potential for a demographic disaster, and health professionals and analysts (e.g. Crewe 1992) were arguing strongly for an integrated AIDS prevention strategy. This finding was subsequently reinforced by the ASSA2000 model. As shown in Figure 2.1, HIV prevalence among pregnant women attending government antenatal clinics rose sharply in the 1990s, as did estimated population HIV-prevalence.

According to Grundlingh (2001), the apartheid South African government's early response to AIDS was 'lukewarm' because of prejudices against homosexuals. Government officials were caught unprepared when the first HIV cases were reported in the heterosexual population, and were hampered by their own 'cultural taboos, ostrich-like complacency, xenophobia, support for a Calvinistic morality and prudishness' (Grundlingh 2001: 28). Unsurprisingly, the apartheid government's belated attempts to promote condom use were denounced as racist and politically motivated. As Ivan Toms (an AIDS activist and anti-apartheid campaigner) said in 1990, 'there is no possibility that the present government could, even if it has the inclination, run an effective campaign to limit the spread of HIV infection. It has no credibility or legitimacy whatsoever among blacks' (quoted in Van der Vliet 2001: 156). If AIDS was to be fought successfully, it was clear that the liberation movements had to be involved.

Fortunately, the African National Congress (ANC) appeared to be taking seriously the possible pandemic. In April 1990 250 delegates, including representatives of the ANC and the pro-ANC United Democratic Front and National Medical and Dental Association, attended a conference on health and welfare in Mozambique. A resolution was drafted encouraging progressive organisations and political leadership to give a leading role to AIDS campaigns within the broader political struggle. This was followed, in 1992, by a conference on AIDS jointly convened by the ANC and the old government's department of health, and attended by a wide range of health professionals, activists and analysts. It represented an 'unusual show of national unity at a time of complex and sensitive political negotiations, well before an election date for a democratically elected government had been decided' (Schneider and Stein 2001: 725). The conference led to the launching of the National AIDS Committee of South Africa (NACOSA), an umbrella body tasked with developing a co-ordinated response to AIDS.

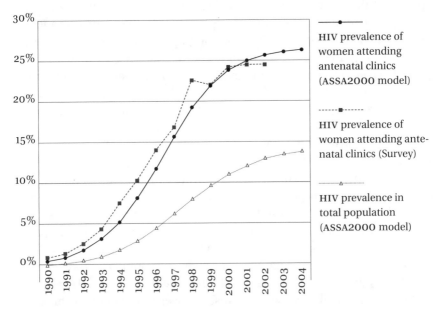

Figure 2.1 *Projections of HIV prevalence from the ASSA2000 demographic model and the antenatal clinic survey (1990–2004)*

The resulting 'AIDS Plan' (developed in September 1993) was comprehens-ive and progressive. As Schneider and Stein point out, 'It went further than the generation of WHO-inspired Medium Term AIDS Plans of the time to embrace the sexual rights of women as a cross cutting theme and to accord people living with AIDS a key role in AIDS policy development and implementation' (2001: 725). It proposed a multi-sectoral structure with implementing units in key ministries (health, welfare, education, defence), but with ultimate responsibility for co-ordination lying with the national president's office. It is worth noting that two of the eight-member drafting team would go on to become consecutive health ministers in the new South African government: Dr Nkosazana Dlamini-Zuma and Dr Manto Tshabalala-Msimang (Van der Vliet 2001: 160).

But while progressive policy was being formulated through such initi-atives, the response by political activists and trade unionists was relatively disappointing since political and organisational imperatives effectively marginalised the AIDS agenda (Crewe 1992; Marais 2000; Van der Vliet 2001). It is possible that AIDS might have been downplayed in order to ease the assimilation of returning exiles, many of whom were returning from high HIV-prevalence areas (Marais 2000: 45). But, whatever the reason, it is clear that the transitional period of the early 1990s was not a conducive environment for addressing AIDS and contributed to the rapid spread of HIV.

When the government of national unity (led by the ANC) took over the reigns of power in 1994, one of its first steps was to adopt the AIDS Plan. In addition, AIDS was declared a 'presidential lead project', giving it preferen-tial access to funds. A National AIDS Programme Director was appointed in December – and it was at this point that the AIDS initiative veered away from the direction outlined in the AIDS Plan and subsequently lost strength and focus.

An important aspect of the problem was that the AIDS Programme Director was placed in the department of health, rather than in the president's office. Provincial governments followed suit by placing responsibility for AIDS programmes in their health ministries. This had the effect of recasting AIDS as a health (rather than a social) problem, and limiting the potential for a multi-sectoral co-ordinated response. Schneider and Stein argue that a further problem with the strategy was that the provincial-level AIDS managers were drawn at fairly low levels of seniority from the ranks of the old civil service and were given the task of imple-menting a programme through weak district structures over which they had no direct line of authority (2001: 726). Marais points to power struggles between officials at different levels of government as a further debilitating factor (2000: 17). The net result was a slow and hesitant start, and an inability on the part of provinces to spend all the money allocated for AIDS, either from the national government or foreign donors.[2]

Could the state have done better? One could certainly hypothesise that if the AIDS Programme Director had been placed in the president's office and if more resources (both human and financial) had been allocated to a vertically and horizontally initiated programme, a better record would probably have emerged. However, as Schneider and Stein observe, such a strategy would still have fallen foul of infrastructural problems at provincial and district level. They argue that the AIDS Plan seriously overestimated the implementation capacity of the transitional government (2001: 726).

But this can never be an entirely adequate excuse for government failure: if infrastructural limitations were the problem, then why did the state not act faster to eliminate them? One (increasingly tired) explanation is to point fingers at the 'inherited' bureaucracy, and blame the difficulties involved in trying to amalgamate the many apartheid bureaucracies into a more efficient system. The old apartheid system had divided the country into a patchwork of provinces, 'independent Bantustans' and African 'homelands'. After the democratic transition, the Bantustans and homelands were absorbed into (restructured) self-governing provinces with financial responsibilities for key functions including health, welfare and education. The process of bureaucratic restructuring and ensuring greater equity in spending between the different regions was certainly difficult and impeded progress in health, education and welfare policy reform. But pointing to such difficulties as a reason for the failure to deliver an adequate public health response is credible only for so long. There is a limit to how long a government can blame its own bureaucracy without being held to account for that failure.

Instead of acting quickly and efficiently to solve the implementation problems, South Africa's political leadership initially engaged in disastrous high profile 'quick-fix' solutions. When these failed, and as HIV prevalence increased, the government went on the defensive by questioning the cost-effectiveness and affordability of AIDS interventions requiring the use of antiretrovirals.

Disastrous high-profile quick-fix solutions

According to Schneider and Stein, the various high-profile scandals concerning AIDS policy in South Africa were 'precipitated by centralised actions of politicians suggesting that they, in fact, were under pressure to act on AIDS, and were searching for short-term solutions' (2001: 727). The first such high-profile controversy began in 1995 when a decision was made at ministerial level to commission *Sarafina II*. The idea was to produce a stage sequel to the popular film musical *Sarafina*, and to give it a distinct anti-AIDS message. A contract of R14.2 million was signed with the playwright and production started.

But while the idea of using popular culture as a medium for reaching young people was innovative, the entire process was rushed and flawed. Firstly, there was no consultation with AIDS experts and activists about how the anti-AIDS message could best be portrayed in a play (Van der Vliet 2001: 162–3). When the play began, the script was widely panned as confused and irrelevant. Secondly, the government failed to comply with its own tender procedures and failed to get permission to spend this large sum of money from the European Union (whose funds were being used for the project). The public outcry over *Sarafina II* resulted in an investigation by the Public Protector and in the subsequent cancellation of the contract.

The *Sarafina II* scandal was incredibly damaging to the government: 'For months, *Sarafina II* represented the public face not only of the AIDS programme, but also of the health department generally. President Mandela, in a review of 1996, cited it as one of the ANC's key mistakes of the year' (Schneider and Stein 2001: 728). It also represented what Van der Vliet describes as a 'watershed event in the relations between the government and civil society' (2001: 163). She quotes a NACOSA briefing to the parliamentary portfolio committee on health:

Sarafina II has done immense damage to individuals and organisations active in the AIDS field. The process was not transparent and this has resulted in a rift between the Department of Health, NACOSA and the NGOs, as well as public derision about and hostility to HIV/AIDS work and programmes (ibid.).

Unfortunately the government did not seem to learn the lesson that quick-fix solutions were not the way forward. Soon thereafter, in February 1997, a cabinet press release announced the development of 'Virodene', a South African treatment for AIDS. Virodene turned out to be an industrial solvent (dimethylformamide) that had previously been tested in cancer therapy but had been abandoned as ineffective and toxic. It had been proposed by a small team of researchers at the University of Pretoria who had administered it to a small number of AIDS patients without clearing its use via the normal ethical and scientific protocols. They managed to obtain an audience with the cabinet, justifying this unusual (indeed extraordinary) step on the grounds that 'the AIDS establishment' was blocking their research because it threatened their patents (Van der Vliet 2001: 164).

The scandal around Virodene persisted for almost a year amid allegations of the government's financial involvement, repeated rejections of Virodene by the Medicines Control Council (MCC), and appeals from people living with AIDS to release the treatment for use. This episode was tragic in that it falsely raised the hopes of people living with AIDS, and further mired South Africa's AIDS initiative in controversy (Crewe 1998). Instead of emerging victorious with a new African miracle cure, the government's reputation was harmed by the strong aroma of sleaze which permeated the Virodene episode, and by the fact that it ignored scientific checks and balances. Instead of accepting the recommendations of the MCC, the government undermined the body by removing the chairperson and replacing him (and others) with more compliant members.

The cabinet's involvement in the Virodene scandal marked another turning point in South African AIDS policy making: the apparent questioning of the science of HIV and AIDS treatment by senior politicians. Once the ANC obtained full power (after the collapse of the government of national unity), and especially after Thabo Mbeki became state president (in June 1999), government policy making became increasingly centralised. This meant that ill-advised views and positions on AIDS, if held by influential politicians such as the minister of health, but especially the state president, had a major impact on policy formulation. It also had an impact on public medical bodies like the MCC and the Medical Research Council – both of which were subjected to thinly veiled purges of those who resisted the government's views on AIDS and AIDS treatment.

The strong influence of Mbeki's ideology over policy making is partly a product of a style of leadership that was developed during the ANC's long years of exile and armed struggle against apartheid.[3] Mbeki's response to a potential leadership challenge in 2001 from three senior ANC members (Sexwale, Phosa and Ramaphosa) was reminiscent of the militaristic and often paranoid years when the ANC was a liberation movement. Rather than engage his challengers in a democratic power struggle, Mbeki launched a police enquiry and accused them of 'plotting' against him. Although no charges were brought against the three men (and the minister for safety and security was forced to apologise to them in public), the episode sent a clear message to other potential leadership challengers that their task would not be easy. A similarly intolerant approach is evident on the part of Mbeki and the cabinet towards criticism of AIDS policy by civil society. High-ranking civil servants in the ministry of health routinely present themselves as being trapped between civil society and their impetuous political masters, and warn activists and medical practitioners not to 'offend' the politicians and to be 'constructive'.[4] Whether intentional or not, the impression is created of a political leadership so concerned about status that it is prepared to act out of pique when criticised. This rather infantile approach to political debate and civil society mobilisation does not bode well for democracy or the rational resolution of AIDS policy debates.

Mbeki's hold on policy making is also a product of South Africa's post-apartheid system of proportional representation. Those towards the top of the ANC's election list are guaranteed their seats, whereas those towards the bottom are not. Under these conditions, there is little incentive for ANC politicians to question, or at least to be seen to be questioning, the views of the political leadership because it is the leadership that deter-mines the order of names on the list. Internal ANC debate is thus muted, as are the prospects for democratically driven shifts in ANC policy.

The discourse of unaffordability of mother-to-child transmission prevention

In October 1998 the health minister (Dlamini-Zuma) announced that South Africa would not be making Zidovudine (AZT) available for MTCTP, and that all planned pilot projects were to be discontinued. Responding to criticism, she said: 'AZT treatment will have a limited effect on the epidemic, as we are targeting individuals already infected' (quoted in Van der Vliet 2001: 167). Comments such as these suggest that the government regarded all use of antiretrovirals as 'treatment', when in the case of MTCTP their use is explicitly connected to prevention (of HIV infection of infants).

In justifying the decision not to introduce MTCTP, national government officials argued that the costs of testing all pregnant women for the virus, of providing the necessary counselling, and of supplying infant formula (to prevent transmission of HIV through breast milk) were too high (Van der Vliet 2001: 166–7). The health ministry persisted with this discourse of unaffordability despite medical and economic research showing that the costs of MTCTP were more than offset by the cost-savings associated with reduced numbers of HIV-related paediatric cases (Nattrass 1998a; McIntyre and Gray 1999; Söderland *et al.* 1999; Wilkinson *et al.* 2000; Geffen 2000; Hensher 2000; Skordis 2000). Nono Simelela, chief director (HIV/AIDS and STDs) in the department of health, argued in the *Mail and Guardian* (28 July to 3 August 2000) that those advocating MTCTP programmes were 'cherry-picking' and that this was a 'luxury' that the health ministry could not afford as it had to respond to the health needs of all South Africans. In other words, the concern was that money spent on MTCTP was money lost to other parts of the health sector.

The health ministry's intransigence unleashed a storm of protest from researchers, AIDS activists and church leaders. In early 2001, the national government appeared to be changing its stance and announced that selected hospitals would provide free HIV tests to pregnant women. Those who tested positive would be offered a short course of Nevirapine and six months' supply of infant formula. This apparent concession, however, was not put into practice at national level, and the decision was referred back to cabinet. In July 2001, TAC instigated legal proceedings against the government to force it to implement a national MTCTP programme. As discussed in Chapter 3, the director general of health (Dr Ayanda Ntsaluba) argued in his replying affidavit that MTCTP was unaffordable and would put too many strains on the health service. The Constitutional Court disagreed and ruled in favour of TAC.

The government eventually started rolling out a national MTCTP programme, but only after being obliged to do so by the Constitutional Court ruling. With the exception of Mpumulanga (where TAC was forced to pursue contempt of court charges against the MEC for health), most provinces took steps to provide pregnant women with access to MTCTP interventions – although with varying degrees of commitment and success. According to a report in the *Mail and Guardian,* South Africa's MTCTP programme in mid-2003 was still a 'shambles' in all provinces except for the Western Cape, Gauteng and KwaZulu-Natal (27 June to 3 July 2003). TAC's strategy is now to force a faster, better and more comprehensive roll-out of both MTCTP and HAART programmes in the public health sector.

Questioning the science of AIDS

Just as the cabinet disregarded scientific evidence and protocols in the Virodene saga, the health minister's position on MTCTP flew in the face of the established and growing body of scientific evidence that a short-course of antiretroviral medication was an effective means of saving lives (see Chapter 3). Not only was the national government's position at odds with medical and economic research, but it was at odds with medical professionals working in public hospitals and with the Western Cape provincial government. In January 1999, the Western Cape provincial government (which was not controlled by the ANC at the time) decided to ignore the national policy and went ahead with MTCTP pilot projects in poor communities with high levels of HIV-infection. They were joined in this effort by Médecins Sans Frontières (MSF).

After the 1999 election, Dlamini-Zuma was redeployed as minister of foreign affairs, and Dr Manto Tshabalala-Msimang became minister of health. Her appointment initially generated optimism, especially after her trip to Uganda to review their AIDS programmes, including recent MTCTP projects. In her first press conference in June 1999, Tshabalala-Msimang said that she was examining ways of ensuring a sustainable AZT programme for MTCTP (Van der Vliet 2001: 168). However, hope soon evaporated when the new president (Thabo Mbeki) made the first of his public interventions in the debate about antiretrovirals. In an address to the National Council of Provinces, he pointed to the problem of toxicity regarding AZT, and asked the health minister to find out where 'the truth lies'. He also urged council members to consult 'the huge volume of literature on this matter available on the Internet' (cited in Van der Vliet 2001: 169). In his own forays into cyberspace, Mbeki appears to have been impressed by websites such as virusmyth.com, where a small network of AIDS dissidents publish alternative (discredited) theories about AIDS.[5] These include the proposition that HIV is a harmless passenger virus and that the symptoms associated with AIDS are the result of poverty and lifestyle choices – and even the result of antiretroviral medication.

The intervention of the president into the AIDS debate appears to have altered Tshabalala-Msimang's stance. Despite the fact that AZT was on the World Health Organisation's list of essential drugs, had been endorsed by South Africa's MCC and by the US Food and Drug Administration and Centres for Disease Control, she was later quoted as saying that AZT weakened the immune system and could lead to 'mutations' and birth defects (Van der Vliet 2001: 169). Like the state president, it appeared she was effectively downgrading established scientific opinion and protocol-approved treatment to the status of being just one among many views.

This, of course, made it impossible to follow scientific principles in adjudicating between rival theories. By giving dissident websites equal status with the MCC, South Africa's political leadership propelled AIDS policy making into a scientific dark age. Under these conditions, 'true statements' could not be established and, in the end, policy making was determined by power. Initially that power vested entirely with the state president. Only when TAC used the courts to contest health policy, was this power eroded to any extent. The constitutional court victory indicated that there were limits to presidential power if/when the exercise thereof entailed a violation of the constitution.

AIDS policy in 2000 was characterised by the political marginalisation of established scientific information and modes of discourse. In January the South African National AIDS Council (SANAC) was launched, but, instead of being the envisaged council of experts, it contained no scientists, no medical practitioners, no representatives from the Medical Research Council or the MCC, and no representatives from high-profile civil society groups like TAC or the AIDS Law Project. This body was not only unrepresentative but also ineffective. When, two years later, Richard Feachem from the Global Fund for HIV/AIDS, TB and Malaria visited South Africa to evaluate SANAC, he concluded that 'it is not yet functional' and 'does not meet often enough and do concrete work' (reported in the *Mail and Guardian*, 11–17 April 2003). It thus appeared to have been set up as a lame duck and behaved as such.

Shortly after the launch of SANAC, President Mbeki created the 'Presidential International Panel of Scientists of HIV in Africa', containing conventional scientists and dissidents (who believed that AIDS was caused by poverty rather than HIV) to explore 'all aspects of the challenge of developing prevention and treatment strategies that are appropriate to the African reality'. The health ministry noted that the inclusion of AIDS dissidents had 'caused uproar among the scientific and medical fraternity', but justified this on the grounds that 'blind acceptance of conventional wisdom would be irresponsible' (cited in Van der Vliet 2001: 171). Thabo Mbeki repeatedly emphasised (including in letters to the UN secretary general, the British prime minister and the US president) that the search for targeted responses to the specifically African nature of the pandemic required an innovative approach, which *inter alia* entailed taking dissident opinions seriously.

The ANC followed suit. On 22 March 2002, the National Executive Committee released a statement supporting the ongoing work of the Presidential Panel:

[W]e will not be stampeded into precipitate action by pseudo-science, an uncaring drive for profits or an opportunistic clamour for cheap popularity ... [W]e shall combat populism, and opportunism that derives from cheap politicking or from benefits lavished by the lobby of powerful local and international interests (ANC 2002).

Thabo Mbeki's interventions in the AIDS debate resulted in widespread confusion. As Judge Edwin Cameron (himself HIV-positive) put it when he addressed the Durban AIDS conference in 2000, Mbeki's

flirtation with those who in the face of all reason and evidence have sought to dispute the etiology of AIDS ... has shaken almost everyone responsible for engaging the epidemic. It has created an air of unbelief amongst scientists, confusion amongst those at risk of HIV, and consternation amongst AIDS workers (Cameron 2000).

Whether Mbeki was simply pointing to the importance of understanding poverty as a key determinant of HIV transmission or actually adopting a dissident/denialist position is an open question. His verbal gymnastics and failure to clarify his position on the causal connection between HIV and AIDS were not helpful. As Crewe points out:

Public questioning of AIDS knowledge has reinforced the doubts and denial that have caused society's lack of behaviour change. If, as the dissidents claim, HIV neither causes AIDS nor is infectious, then the safe sex message of responsible sexual decision-making, issues of gender and of domestic violence, and recognition of the seriousness of the epidemic, fall away. Vexing questions of culture, race and sexual behaviour need not be addressed. It is unnecessary to deal with patterns of male sexual behaviour, and with gender imbalances in vulnerability to infection. It is no longer imperative to change people's attitudes so as to bring about changes in behaviour. HIV infection now will be seen as the 'logical' outcome of poverty, malnutrition and poor socio-economic conditions, and there is very little government can, or need do, to try and combat it (2000: 25–6).

Mbeki's questioning of established scientific knowledge and best-practice medical interventions succeeded in driving a wedge between the scientific community and the government. Professor Hoosen Coovadia, chairperson of the AIDS 2000 Conference, and two colleagues made a public plea for Mbeki to keep clear of the scientific debates. This was met with an aggressive response by three cabinet ministers, who accused Coovadia and his colleagues of being 'journeymen rather than geniuses', saying that they would never be satisfied with 'anything short of provision of antiretrovirals in the public health system'. They concluded: 'here we draw a clear line between informed and responsible recommendations on therapeutic interventions by scientists, and standing out as the frontline troops for the pharmaceutical industry' (cited in Van der Vliet 2001: 174).

Distrust of the pharmaceutical companies is a common thread running though many official government pronouncements on AIDS policy. For example, in response to a letter from the head of the Methodist Church, a high court judge, the Anglican archbishop, and the chairperson of the AIDS 2000 conference appealing for the provision of AZT to pregnant HIV-positive women, Mbeki had the following to say:

I am taken aback by the determination of many people in our country to sacrifice all intellectual integrity to act as salespersons of the product of one pharmaceutical company (cited in Van der Vliet 2001: 174).

As this kind of argument is typical of AIDS dissidents, its main effect was to cast Mbeki further in the role of a dissident. After all, if the problem is one of price and excess profits, the appropriate response would be to follow the lead of other developing countries and negotiate with the large pharmaceutical companies for bulk discounts (perhaps within the framework of the United Nations' Accelerated Access Initiative), or to consider ways of accessing (or even producing) bulk generics. Instead, the response, as couched by Mbeki, was designed more to discredit those who argued in favour of using antiretrovirals.

The way the government handled the high-profile court case brought against it by the Pharmaceutical Manufacturers' Association (PMA) is informative. In 1997 the government passed the Medicines and Related Substances Control Amendment Act, which, although ambiguous, appeared to give the minister of health wide powers to facilitate parallel importation[6] and compulsory licensing[7] of essential drugs. The PMA challenged the constitutionality of the Act, saying that it contravened South Africa's obligations as a member of the World Trade Organisation. The PMA was particularly concerned about the possibility of compulsory licensing (Cleary and Ross 2002). The South African government refused to back down on the issue in subsequent negotiations. The case came to court in March 2001, at which point TAC was admitted by the Court as *amicus curiae* (friend of the court). This caused the proceedings to be delayed by a month, and when the case was reopened in April the PMA immediately offered to settle the case and the government accepted.

The government hailed the settlement as a 'historic victory' and this view was reflected in the local and international media. However, as Cleary and Ross (2002) point out, the settlement in fact conceded the very issue the PMA went to court over, namely compulsory licensing. In the out-of-court settlement, the government agreed to rephrase parts of the Act to make it clear that compulsory licensing was *not* being provided for. Cleary and Ross explain this outcome on the grounds that the South African government had changed its position between 1997 and 2001 – largely because AIDS activists had succeeded in portraying the court case as being about access to antiretrovirals (2002: 454). According to Cleary and Ross (2002), this resulted in the South African government no longer wanting to win the case – and thus being prepared to settle out of court. The main benefit to the PMA (aside from effectively winning the case) was that by settling out of court they avoided having to present evidence about how much profit they had already made out of AIDS drugs:

We conclude that the success of HIV/AIDS activists in publicly spinning the original court case as a battle over access to HIV/AIDS therapies complicated the game for both the South African Government and the PMA. The resulting threat of rising public demonisation increased the cost to the PMA of pursuing its suit, especially as enhanced legal and public scrutiny would likely have revealed the extent of its already achieved profits from HIV/AIDS drugs. At the same time, the value to the Government of securing the right to compulsory licensing diminished, given the conflict between this goal and its desire not to become responsible for antiretroviral provision under *any* legal regime (Cleary and Ross 2002: 489–90; emphasis in the original).

Cleary and Ross hypothesise that this shift in the government's 'utility function' was rational. While admitting that irrational factors (such as Mbeki's dissident views) may have played a role, they show that a rational interpretation can be placed on the government's change in policy stance. The reasons they give for why a 'rational' South African government may have backed away from compulsory licensing include wanting to appear to be a 'model citizen' in the World Trade Organisation and not wanting to undermine its policy of fiscal restraint by appearing to be conceding ground on the AIDS treatment issue. On the latter point, Cleary and Ross argue that it is reasonable 'to suppose that the Government would prefer – relative to some unknown maximum level of commitment to humanitarian concerns – to minimise its fiscal exposure to the potentially enormous costs of direct state responsibility for provision of palliative treatment to victims of the expanding HIV/AIDS epidemic' (2002: 456).

Whether the government's hostility to antiretroviral interventions was in some narrow sense economically rational (in the way described by Cleary and Ross), or whether it is best explained with reference to the Mbeki presidency, is ultimately an empirical issue. According to Schneider, the dispute between President Mbeki (and his acolytes) and the 'AIDS world' should be seen as a struggle over symbolic power: 'Ultimately, policy contestation around AIDS in South Africa can be understood as a series of attempts by the state to legitimately define who has the right to speak about AIDS, to determine the response to AIDS and even to define the problem itself' (2001: 10). Such an analysis, however, begs the question of whether the power struggle was simply symbolic – or whether there is a material basis for it. Nevertheless, it is clear that since October 2000, when Thabo Mbeki announced that he was withdrawing from the public debate about the science of AIDS, the argument against antiretroviral provision has been increasingly couched in economic terms.

Since April 2001, when the cabinet released a statement to the effect that HIV causes AIDS, South African policy making has supposedly been conducted 'on the assumption that HIV causes AIDS'. According to Jacobs and Calland, the key moment for Mbeki occurred in April 2002 when the Canadian president, Jean Chretien, visited South Africa. Mbeki agreed to be interviewed by Canadian journalists, ostensibly on the subject of the New Partnership for Africa's Development (NEPAD), but was instead subjected to a barrage of questions about AIDS:

Whether or not this represented some kind of epiphanous moment, or was simply the straw that broke the camel's back, is unclear. It does seem, however, that the penny finally dropped for Mbeki: his views on HIV/AIDS were destroying not only his international reputation, but the credibility of the entire NEPAD project. That it should take him so long to reach this understanding is an indictment not just of his advisers' failure to persuade him of the seriousness of the situation, but of his lack of political wit (2002: 4).

Although Mbeki effectively bowed out of the AIDS debate, the 'dead-hand of denialism' (Cameron 2003: 4) seemed to weigh on AIDS policy formation through 2002 and into 2003. For example, in January 2003, presidential spokesperson Smuts Ngongyama was quoted as saying that the importation of Brazilian generic antiretrovirals (by MSF) amounted to 'biological warfare' (*The Star*, 31 January 2003).[8] That same month, Tshabalala-Msimang invited Robert Giraldo, a prominent AIDS denialist, to address the Southern Africa Development Community Ministerial

Health Committee. Giraldo informed the committee that 'the transmission of AIDS from person to person is a myth' and that 'the heterosexual transmission in Africa is an assumption made without any scientific validation' (cited in Cameron 2003: 2). Giraldo was subsequently invited by Tshabala-Msimang to advise the South African government about nutrition. Given this context, it is understandable why, in August 2003, when the cabinet accepted that 'antiretroviral drugs do help improve the quality of life of those at a certain stage of the development of AIDS', it was greeted with such widespread jubilation and relief (*Sunday Independent,* 9 August 2003).

The cabinet statement in support of antiretroviral treatment was, in fact, very cautious and highly qualified. Rather than agreeing to allow the many hospitals (and other medical sites) with adequate capacity to start implementing antiretroviral treatment as soon as possible, the cabinet asked the department of health to develop a detailed operational plan. This unnecessary delay to the start of the treatment roll-out was consistent with the government's emerging discourse of the complexity of AIDS treatment interventions, and the necessity to conduct exhaustive planning before any treatment could be provided anywhere in the public health system. Problems of drug resistance, toxicity, patient adherence to drug regimens and infrastructure requirements were highlighted along with the need to ensure that any treatment programme had to be 'sustainable' – i.e. sufficient resources had to be available over the long term to support the programme. This clearly puts the spotlight straight onto the issue of affordability.

The discourse of unaffordability of AIDS treatment

The AIDS policy debate in 2003 was focussed on the feasibility, affordability and implementation of a national treatment plan. In February, the health minister refused to sign the 'framework agreement' on AIDS treatment which had been negotiated in NEDLAC by representatives of labour, business, government and civil society, citing cost factors and implementation complexities (*Mail and Guardian,* 21–27 February 2003). The matter was referred to a Joint Health and Treasury Task Team (JHTTT) for costing.

The following week the minister explained her position more fully in a newspaper article, arguing that the government was waiting for the results of the task team into the costs of procuring and dispensing antiretrovirals before making a decision about how to proceed on the issue. Given that there were several other substantial costing exercises already in the public domain (see review by Boulle *et al.* 2003), the need for this exercise was far from clear. The exercise was thus widely perceived in the AIDS advocacy arena as yet another government delaying tactic. At the time, however, the health minister sought to dispel such an impression. She wrote:

I want to state quite plainly that we are concerned about the challenges that HIV and AIDS treatment poses. We are not trying to dodge the issues but to come to terms with their complexities. We want to offer the best this country can – and do so in a sustainable manner that overcomes many of the weaknesses in our delivery systems ... The fact that this government places the challenge of poverty squarely on the AIDS agenda is not an indication that we are reluctant to tackle the issues of treatment. Quite the opposite: poverty eradication and medical interventions are mutually reinforcing and we would be selling our people short if we did not attend to both (*Mail and Guardian,* 28 February to 6 March 2003).

The concern about sustainability/affordability remained on the policy agenda throughout 2003. The Joint Health and Treasury Task Team investigated the costs of a treatment roll-out and reported to cabinet in May. In August the cabinet noted the contents of the report, pronounced support in principle for AIDS treatment, but requested a further 'detailed operational plan' in order to 'ensure that the remaining challenges are addressed with urgency; and that the final product guarantees a programme that is effective and sustainable' (cabinet statement, 8 August 2003). The next day the health minister shed light on this rather vague statement by saying 'I can't say we have a roll-out because the plan has not been adequately costed. We are really not happy with the costing yet' (*Mail and Guardian,* 15–21 August 2003).

It seems very likely that the roll-out of AIDS treatment will be dogged by chronic problems relating to costing and resource availability. The cabinet was probably forced into announcing a treatment programme by the sheer weight of public pressure and by concerns to defuse the issue before the 2004 elections. According to a national newspaper, the policy U-turn was the result of a revolt within the cabinet against the state president and the minister of health (*Mail and Guardian,* 15–21 August 2003). If so, it was a very incomplete coup. The minister of health remained in her post and continues to dictate the scale and pace of the treatment roll-out. Furthermore, other signals emanating from the government also reflect a deep reluctance to allocate significant resources to such an intervention. Shortly after his 2003/4 budget speech (which announced a significant increase in the allocation for combating AIDS), the finance minister argued that the bulk of expenditure on AIDS should be on prevention rather than treatment and that provincial governments should spend their money on other priorities, such as education, rather than antiretrovirals (*Business Day*, 19 March 2003). In other words, at least in the mind of the finance minister – who after all has the greatest effective say in resource allocation – antiretroviral treatment was not a priority. As argued below, the government's explicit and implicit position on AIDS treatment amounts to a 'moral economy of triage'.

2.2 The moral economy of triage

The concept of triage rose to prominence in field hospitals in the Crimean War, where doctors were confronted by a huge and immediate imbalance between the numbers of people needing medical attention and the limited resources available for the job. So they divided the wounded soldiers into three groups: those who would probably recover without treatment; those with a good chance of recovery if they received attention; and those with little hope of surviving even if they were given treatment. Resources were then allocated first to those with good prospects of recovery if they obtained treatment, and last (if at all) to the very badly wounded – the objective being to save as many lives as possible with the limited resources available.

Triage was both rational (it made optimal use of resources) and reasonable in the sense that reasonable citizens would agree that it was appropriate under the circumstances. Triage is reasonable in extreme situations where two conditions exist: (1) resources are absolutely constrained, and (2) the allocation of resources is a zero-sum game. According to Marseille *et al.*, triage is an appropriate way for developing countries to respond to the AIDS pandemic:

The classic situation occurs in wartime and natural disasters in which a triage process determines how limited resources will be allocated. Now, for perhaps the first time in history, we must decide whether economic reality will permit an informed debate about rationing that could result in millions of patients receiving supportive care, but not treatment, to prevent many more millions from becoming afflicted with the disease. The allocation of resources, the development of a just health-care system and the adjudication of the rights and claims of competing groups 'are and will be the important moral problems of the future'. Indeed these are the present moral issues facing HIV policy-makers in sub-Saharan Africa (2002: 1855).

The South African government seems to agree with this prognosis. Since the late 1990s, the dominant theme on the subject, as espoused by the state president and the ministers of health and finance, was that South Africa 'could not afford' to provide HAART because the drug costs were 'prohibitive' and the administrative requirements 'too complex'. In 2003, as it became clear that some kind of treatment intervention had to be announced for political reasons, the government's discourse shifted to the more subtle argument that AIDS treatment interventions must be 'sustainable' – i.e. constrained by available resources. But this, of course, begs the question of the level of available resources. As noted above, the minister of finance argues that South Africa should concentrate on preventing new HIV-infections and on pursuing social objectives (like building schools), rather than spending money on prolonging the life of people with AIDS. The choice is presented in classic triage terms: we have scarce resources; HIV-positive people cannot be cured; therefore, instead of devoting significant resources to prolonging their lives through treatment, we should save the lives of others (through prevention) and otherwise concentrate on developmental goals.

There is, however, a serious problem with the triage metaphor when applied to AIDS policy: the allocation of resources between HAART and prevention is *not* a zero-sum game. Treatment programmes can have a strong preventive impact (Chapters 4 and 5). Rather than looking myopically at individual cases needing immediate treatment, policy makers should be thinking about the impact on total resource costs over time. This will be affected by fewer HIV infections and lower AIDS-related morbidity and mortality resulting from treatment.

As argued in Chapter 3, an MTCTP programme in South Africa will almost certainly pay for itself by reducing the flow of AIDS-related paediatric cases to government health facilities. Chapter 4 takes the argument further, and shows that the cost savings to the government (in terms of lower AIDS morbidity and fewer new HIV infections associated with a HAART programme) reduce the overall health sector costs substantially. Average cost per AIDS death averted is lower for an AIDS intervention that includes HAART than it is for one that does not.

One response to this is to point out that this analysis assumes that the resources are available for the large-scale AIDS intervention including treatment. What if very few resources are available? Under such conditions, we need to know what the marginal costs and benefits are of moving from prevention-only interventions, to a broader intervention that includes HAART. This is, of course, entirely correct. But it brings us to the second problem with the Crimean field hospital analogy, i.e. the assumption of absolutely limited supplies and no hope of replenishing them while the fighting lasts. The health budget, like any other budget, is obviously limited by available social resources, but the size of each budget within this resource envelope is a product of social choice. It is possible that once the overall net costs to the public sector of a large-scale AIDS intervention including treatment are presented to informed citizens for reflection, they will decide to support it. Society may well accept a large increase in the size of the health budget (and in taxation). Appealing to the limited resources in the health sector (or allowing the economic analysis to be framed by it) begs the very question of social choice. We can, in other words, choose to send more supplies to the field hospital. Conversely, we could decide to reallocate resources away from the field hospital and use it to purchase armaments instead. Ultimately, the matter is a question of social values and political power.

The discourse of 'unaffordability' is protected from public scrutiny by what amounts to a technocratic argument on the part of the state that only the government is in a position to evaluate and rank the full spectrum of social objectives/needs/priorities; and that having reviewed all competing claims, has determined that a full-scale roll-out of antiretroviral treatment for all is 'unaffordable'. Many of the infected will thus simply have to die without treatment because resources are supposedly better spent (from a social perspective) on other priorities.

This immediately poses the question: what does the public actually want the government to do about AIDS? Are governments in Southern Africa pulling the wool over everyone's eyes with these kinds of technocratic arguments – or are they acting broadly in line with their own citizens' priorities? Who is the 'we' referred to by Marseille *et al.*, who must decide what is economically feasible and desirable? Or, to use the language of Cleary and Ross (2002: 456), who decides 'the unknown maximum level of commitment to humanitarian concerns' that enters into the government's fiscal calculus concerning HAART?

Stephen Lewis, the United Nations secretary general's special envoy for HIV/AIDS in Africa, has done a great deal to draw international attention to the AIDS crisis in Africa. Writing about a trip he took to Southern Africa, Lewis reported that the issue of anti-retroviral treatment came up constantly and everywhere. Every single group of people living with HIV/AIDS pounded the demand home in unrelenting fashion. There is a crescendo of rage and desperation that governments will ignore at their peril (*Sunday Independent*, 12 January 2003).

Marseille *et al.* are concerned about these protests – but for different reasons, arguing that they are likely to influence politicians and lead to more resources being spent on treatment than is 'optimal' (2002: 1855). Their preferred route is for governments to ignore this rage and make what they assume to be the politically harder choice of promoting prevention-only programmes rather than an intervention that includes HAART. They argue that those whose lives are likely to be saved through prevention interventions are unaware of this benefit, and hence are unlikely to lobby for resources to go towards prevention rather than treatment. This argument amounts to giving technocrats the casting vote because they, unlike the people, know what is best for society.

As already noted, one of the flaws with Marseille *et al.*'s argument is that HAART treatment programmes have a strong preventive element. Treating people with HAART also saves new HIV infections. According to the analysis presented in Chapter 4, expanding an AIDS intervention to include treatment results in a lower average cost for each HIV infection averted. There is thus a case for spending more money on a much bolder set of policies.

Note that this argument is *not* equivalent to saying that the marginal Rand should be moved from prevention to treatment. Such a conclusion can only be drawn from a different kind of study, which takes the budget constraint as given and tries to estimate the 'optimal' allocation of resources (in terms of lives saved) given these constraints. Studies such as these are important and can help advise governments about how best to allocate their budgets.[9] The triage analogy makes sense in this context. But these studies do not, by definition, question the budget constraint. The analysis in Chapter 4 takes a different approach by estimating the total resources required to introduce a large-scale AIDS intervention that includes providing treatment to all those who need it – and then posing the issue of budgetary implications. When the issue is examined from this broader frame of reference, the triage analogy is inappropriate. Triage begs the very question under consideration: how should society respond to the challenges posed by AIDS?

Marseille *et al.*'s position is problematic on democratic grounds as well. The question of whether 'the people' or 'the technocrats' should decide on policy is of fundamental importance. It is, of course, possible that in some cases, ceding decision-making power to technocrats is in the interests of the 'general good'. But for that to be the case, (1) it must be impossible to educate the public about the decision in question and engage citizens in a discussion about social choices, and (2) collective action problems must make it impossible for society to be involved in any sensible decision making process. This book shows that complex economic arguments can be presented clearly (and hence citizens can be educated about choices). Although the government will have to at some level adjudicate between competing claims, it is argued that a social accord process involving representatives of civil society in meaningful dialogue with the government over public policy could bring about more consensus than is commonly assumed. Furthermore, it is contended that the conventional economic wisdom, as espoused by Marseille *et al.*, is not necessarily true – especially with regard to the South African case. Critical discussion about rival economic arguments is thus a desirable component of the process of policy formation.

But what about the second prerequisite? Is it the case that collective action problems make it impossible for society to come to a reasonable and appropriate decision about AIDS policy? According to Marseille *et al.*, if a policy is not directly and obviously in the interests of individuals, they will not lobby for it, and hence – by implication – the outcome will not be socially optimal. Marseille *et al.* worry that the 'Rule of Rescue', which governments often use to allocate resources to identifiable individuals with health needs (e.g. people ill with AIDS), will trump a more rational economic analysis suggesting that the money is better spent on prevention. This is a valid concern, as Paltiel and Stinnett point out:

The Rule of Rescue exerts a powerful force on human intuition. People find it comforting to know that everything possible is being done to save a particular life at risk. We all bask in the joy of rallying together to rescue a toddler from the bottom of a well. A dispassionate analysis might reveal that an equal expenditure could have prevented the deaths of many more children if it were devoted either to building fences around wells or to vaccination programmes and improved automobile safety, but these opportunity costs are measured in faceless statistics and rarely appear on the nightly newscast. They are invisible, and hence, they are easier to ignore. This propensity to tune out the anonymous victim has particular relevance for funding HIV prevention. Epidemic control activities, by their very nature, are aimed at saving 'statistical lives'. Nobody can point with certainty to the particular individual whose life was unequivocally 'saved' by a prevention intervention ... In this sense, the Rule of Rescue gives a comparative advantage to aggressive treatment activities in competing for public sympathy and resources (1998: 144).

Two issues are relevant here. The first has to do with whether the 'Rule of Rescue' features in government decision making, or even in the public imagination, when it comes to considering AIDS treatment interventions in South Africa. Public sympathies are certainly engaged when it comes to rescuing a toddler from a well but it is unlikely that a similar level of sympathy exists for people who are sick with AIDS. This is because treating people with HAART extends rather than saves their lives, and because people living with AIDS may be blamed for their own condition (see Chapter 1). The stigmatisation of AIDS-sufferers is perhaps partly a function of the perception that (as a result of their own sexual choices) they effectively threw themselves down the well. As discussed in Chapter 5, fighting AIDS-related stigma is an important ingredient in any effective strategy to combat the pandemic. Encouraging the public to see people living with AIDS as deserving of 'rescue' is part of the challenge.

The second issue worth considering is the difference between the (individually) rational and the 'reasonable'. To quote Rawls once again, 'rational agents approach being psychopathic when their interests are solely in benefit of themselves' (1993: 51) and that 'in so far as we are reasonable, we are ready to work out the framework for the public social world' (ibid. 53). If we accept that people are in this sense reasonable, then it is plausible to assume that reasonable citizens will be able to grasp both the import of prevention programmes and the importance of the link between treatment and prevention. There is thus no necessary reason why AIDS policy formation should suffer from the kind of collective action problem posed by Marseille *et al.* (2002).

Note, however, that this conclusion depends on there being an adequate forum for public discussion and reflection on important policy issues. If policy making is simply a function of lobbying (as implicitly assumed by Marseille *et al.*), then socially perverse outcomes are not only possible but likely. This highlights the importance of social institutions like NEDLAC to facilitate the involvement of civil society in social and economic policy making. The challenge is to create forums for discussion that include as wide a range of interests as possible. As argued in Chapter 7, there is a need for a broad-based debate on how to address the development dilemma posed by AIDS. The concluding section of this chapter reports on the limited evidence available about existing policy priorities in Southern Africa.

What do Southern African citizens think about policy priorities?

How do the citizens of Southern Africa view policy priorities? Do their views reflect the urgency of addressing AIDS or addressing poverty? Is there a 'crescendo of rage' that threatens political stability? A recent cross-country survey helps shed light on this.

The *Afrobarometer* collected data on political attitudes, socio-economic indicators and various other attitudes (including those on AIDS) in seven Southern African countries between July 1999 and July 2000. The following open-ended question was asked: 'What are the most important problems facing this country that the government should address?' Given the high HIV-prevalence rates among adults in Southern Africa and the large number of AIDS deaths per year (see Table 1.1), one might have expected HIV/AIDS to feature high on the public agenda. However, as indicated in Table 2.1, economic issues – especially job creation – were clearly the top priorities. Only in Zambia did people spontaneously refer to health issues more often than economic issues.

According to Whiteside *et al.*, the relative ranking of HIV/AIDS for government action by *Afrobarometer* respondents did not vary systematically with average country-level HIV-prevalence, the proportion of respondents who knew someone who had died of AIDS, or the number of cumulative deaths from AIDS (2002: 29). They suggest that this could be because economic conditions in Southern Africa are so dire that issues pertaining to immediate income needs were forced to the forefront of people's consciousness. The fact that poorer people were less likely to cite AIDS as a problem than richer people perhaps constitutes evidence for this position (ibid. 31). Whatever the reason, the bottom line is that AIDS and health issues are not, for the most part, perceived as political priorities by the general Southern African population. One could interpret the table as suggesting that the Southern African population agrees with the argument that economic growth and development should be prioritised over direct interventions to treat people living with AIDS. If so, then the South African finance minister is responding to a widely held position in society.

One could, of course, hypothesise that these views are likely to change when death rates rise further. Citizens may then alter their political priorities in favour of health care as the AIDS pandemic continues to reap its

Table 2.1 *Spontaneously reported political priorities in Southern Africa* (Afrobarometer)

Botswana	Zimbabwe	Zambia	Malawi	Lesotho	Namibia	South Africa
Job creation (58%)	Economy (74%)	Health (41%)	Economy (48%)	Job creation (63%)	Job creation (54%)	Job creation (76%)
AIDS (24%)	Job creation (37%)	Job creation (32%)	Health (29%)	Crime/ security (28%)	Education (46%)	Crime/ security (60%)
Education (20%)	Health (18%)	Education (31%)	Crime/ security (28%)	Food (20%)	General services (21%)	Housing (25%)
Poverty and destitution (17%)		Agriculture (26%)	Food (26%)		Health (18%)	Education (13%)
Health (15%)		Economy (20%)	Transport (16%)		AIDS (14%)	AIDS (13%)
Agriculture (14%)		Transport (18%)	Water (16%)			Health (12%)
Crime/ security (12%)		Poverty (14%)	Agriculture (13%)			Poverty (11%)
			Education (12%)			
			Poverty (11%)			
			Job creation (11%)			

Source: Whiteside *et al.* 2002: 30. The table lists only those problems referred to by more than 10% of respondents.

grim harvest. Unfortunately this is impossible to predict – especially given the close relationship between AIDS, poverty and vulnerability. AIDS kills young productive adults, thus plummeting poor households into poverty. Under such conditions, it would hardly be surprising if job creation and welfare were to continue to be prioritised over health expenditure – even by those most devastated by AIDS.

Another way of looking at Table 2.1 is to look at how often AIDS or health-related objectives were mentioned. Rather than judge priorities in terms of whether AIDS/health tops the agenda or not, a more nuanced interpretation would be to ask whether the glass is half full rather than half empty. If Southern African citizens understand that AIDS and development need to be addressed together, then the broad pattern of priorities listed in the table is to be expected. AIDS and health issues feature very high on the agenda. Just because health tops the agenda in only one country does not mean it is not a priority. Indeed, the table could be interpreted as indicating that in spite of the dire development needs of Southern Africa, South African citizens are indicating that something needs to be done now to address health concerns. If most people agreed with the moral economy of triage approach, then one would expect health concerns to feature very low down on the list. The fact that they do not, probably indicates a strong social preference for addressing the health needs of individuals – even if that means diverting resources to them. The question thus boils back down to the development dilemma: what should be done to address health needs, and at what cost to other priorities? This issue is taken up with regard to South Africa in Chapters 6 and 7.

3 Mother-to-child transmission prevention in South Africa

The first major AIDS policy battle in South Africa was over mother-to-child transmission prevention (MTCTP). Between 1998, when the government first pronounced that it would not introduce MTCTP, and 2001, when it was ordered to do so by the constitutional court, the government's position remained implacable: South Africa could not afford it. When questioned by journalists, the minister of health would explain (often with an evident degree of irritation) that South Africa simply did not have the resources. Her implication was clear: people who were demanding such an intervention did not understand economics and were, unlike government officials like herself, not in a position to appreciate the ranking of social priorities.

Chapter 2 touched on a range of factors (including the president's views on antiretrovirals and AIDS) which may have contributed to this inflexible position. This chapter takes the government's argument about affordability at face value, and shows that there is little (if any) basis for it once the costs of *not* introducing MTCTP are considered. The chapter shows that it almost certainly costs the government more to treat the opportunistic infections suffered by HIV-positive children over their short lives than it would to save many of them through MTCTP.

3.1 Introduction

By the late 1990s, there was a wealth of evidence from developed and developing countries that treating pregnant women with a short course of antiretrovirals could dramatically reduce the transmission of HIV from mother to child. South African medical research subsequently came to similar findings (see e.g. Söderland *et al.* 1999; McIntyre and Gray 1999; Wilkinson *et al.* 2000). However, all the recommended treatment regimes entailed the use of HIV tests and antiretrovirals – the very things that President Mbeki was apparently questioning.

This posed a problem for the health ministry because to implement appropriate treatment regimes could have been construed as a slap in the face for the president. But there was another argument against introducing an MTCTP, i.e. that South Africa could 'not afford' it. This argument first reared its head when the health minister (then Nkosazana Zuma) announced in 1998 that antiretrovirals (especially AZT) were too expensive for the government to embark on an MTCTP programme. Arguments to the effect that the paediatric costs of treating the opportunistic infections of HIV-positive children far exceeded the costs of the intervention (see Nattrass 1998a; McIntyre and Gray 1999) appeared to have had no impact. Once the price of AZT was slashed and Nevirapine (a much cheaper but less effective alternative to AZT) was offered free of charge to South Africa for five years, the health ministry's argument lost further credibility. Nevertheless, government officials continued to maintain that the programme was unaffordable. They argued that the costs of testing all pregnant women for HIV, of introducing the necessary counselling services, and of providing infant formula (to prevent transmission of HIV through breast milk) were too high (Van der Vliet 2001: 166–7). The health ministry persisted with this line of argument despite work by economists showing that even after adjusting for these further costs, it was still cost-effective to introduce MTCTP (see Skordis 2000; Geffen 2000; Hensher 2000; Skordis and Nattrass 2002). It eventually took a constitutional court case to force the government to change its policy stance. However, despite the ruling, the government made slow progress in rolling out the programme in any province beyond the Western Cape, Gauteng and KwaZulu-Natal (*Mail and Guardian*, 27 June to 3 July 2003).

The problem with the government's argument is that by concentrating only on additional costs associated with MTCTP, it failed to take account of costs associated with the children who would become HIV-positive in the absence of MTCTP. Such costs have to be taken into account explicitly when evaluating whether the programme is 'affordable' or not.

Methodological considerations

The emerging literature on the cost-effectiveness of MTCTP in South Africa tends to be framed in terms of disability-adjusted-life-years, i.e. DALYs (see e.g. Söderland *et al.* 1999; Geffen 2000; Wilkinson *et al.* 2000). DALYs combine 'time lived with a disability and the time lost due to premature mortality' (Murray 1994: 441). DALYs are age-weighted and include a discount factor.[1]

The DALY is designed to help policy makers rank interventions in terms of cost per DALY saved. But how useful is it when it comes to practical budgetary allocations? In the Wilkinson *et al.* (2000) study, the cost per DALY associated with an AZT-based MTCTP programme was estimated as ranging from $17 (R134) in KwaZulu-Natal to $46 (R369) in the Western Cape (and averaging $27 (R213) nationally).[2] Geffen (2000) estimated (using different assumptions about formula feeding, seroprevalence and other variables) that the national cost per DALY of an AZT regime to reduce mother-to-child transmission was almost three times higher, at $76 (R606) per DALY.

While such calculations are an interesting first step, they are only really meaningful from a policy perspective when placed in the context of a range of costs per DALY for different interventions. These must include not only interventions in the health sector, but also all other government programmes and projects that improve health indicators (e.g. the provision of clean water, the removal of environmental hazards, income-generating programmes, etc.). As Anand and Hanson point out:

> If mothers' education, or improving water supply and sanitation conditions generate bigger 'bang-for-a-buck' than health interventions, then the health budget should be redirected to the ministry of education, or of public utilities. A committed DALY maximiser should in principle be willing to give over this entire health budget to other ministries! Otherwise, his restricted cost-effectiveness exercise can lead to a seriously suboptimal allocation of resources in the improvement of health outcomes (1997: 699).

In South Africa's case, very few DALY calculations have been made with regard to government programmes. Wilkinson *et al.* (2000) report two other estimates for comparative purposes: an immunisation programme ranging from $25–30 per DALY, and a family planning programme at $100–150 per DALY (both in 1990 prices). But what does this mean in policy terms? Does it mean that we should be putting more money into MTCTP than into family planning? And, given that immunisation appears to be more cost-effective than MTCTP in the Western Cape, should we put money into the former rather than the latter programme? Of course Wilkinson *et al.* (2000) would argue against any such interpretation as there are no doubt many other programmes (such as kidney dialysis and heart transplants) that are undoubtedly much less cost-effective in terms of cost per DALY. However, until such time as a significant number of comparable DALY studies (using similar assumptions) have been done, an isolated cost-effectiveness measure (or even a small collection of such measures) is of limited policy significance.[3]

Some South African authors have attempted to get around this problem by comparing cost per DALY to some kind of objective standard of cost-effectiveness. For example, Söderlund *et al.* (1999) suggest that interventions costing less than $100 per life year saved are cost-effective for developing countries. Geffen (2000) uses the same figure as a benchmark to argue that MTCTP is cost-effective, and hence worth doing. Scholars working on data from other African countries also rely on benchmarking. For example, Stringer *et al.* (2000) opt for $50 a life year saved when evaluating the cost-effectiveness of MTCTP in sub-Saharan Africa. Most international cost-effectiveness studies end up comparing their DALY estimates with such benchmarks (Creese *et al.* 2002).

The problem with this kind of analysis is that it is arbitrary (on what basis should we pick $50 over $100, or any other figure for that matter?) and runs counter to the original purpose of the DALY as a tool for allocating health resources between competing claims. It begs the question of how many *other* interventions cost less than $50 or $100 per DALY and fails to interrogate the problem of using a rough international indicator as a benchmark against which to evaluate policies at country level. At most, presenting such cost-effectiveness calculations alongside an international benchmark provides only a rough indication that the cost per (adjusted) life year is in some sense low.

In the absence of any means to rank the cost per DALY in terms of the cost-effectiveness of alternative interventions, the existing South African studies express the total costs of the programme as a percentage of the health budget in order to show the relatively limited resource implications of the intervention. Wilkinson *et al.* (2000) report that a national MTCTP programme would amount to less than 1% of the national health budget – or $0.49 per person living in South Africa. In his review of the available studies, Geffen observes that there is consensus in the South African literature that such a programme will not cost more than 3% of the national government health budget (2000: 5).

But while this is more helpful to the process of budgetary allocation than a raw cost per DALY, it is not sufficient. The calculation outlined below takes the argument one step further by comparing the costs of the programme with the costs associated with *not* making the intervention. It starts with a 'base-line' estimate of the cost to the health sector of not introducing MTCTP. This is followed by an estimate of the cost-effectiveness of introducing a short-course AZT regimen and a short-course Nevirapine regimen – both with and without substitute feeding. The analysis is an updated and extended version of Nattrass (2001a). It is presented in 2001 prices and includes a sensitivity analysis which varies key costs by 25%. This alternative approach to affordability does not entail the use of DALYs, and does not require comparison with any benchmark 'cost per DALY' to arrive at the policy conclusion. A similar DALY-free approach is adopted in Chapter 4, which considers a full range of AIDS prevention and treatment interventions.

3.2 Why South Africa cannot *not* afford mother-to-child transmission prevention

In order to address this question, it is helpful to start with a 'base-line' scenario of the costs of not introducing MTCTP, and then to compare it with the total costs to the health sector of MTCTP. The full costing exercise is provided in the appendix to this chapter. In order to simplify the argument, the analysis is presented in terms of the health costs associated with (a hypothetical random sample of) 1,000 pregnant women attending antenatal clinics in South Africa.

According to antenatal survey data, for every 1,000 pregnant women visiting government clinics, 24.5% will be HIV-positive. Of these 245 women, 30% will transmit the virus to their babies (either through the birth process, or through subsequent breastfeeding) if no MTCTP programme is available. This means that 74 children will be born HIV-positive in the normal course of events. These HIV-positive children will suffer from opportunistic infections during their short lives and will require treatment. The best-estimate calculation is based on information from the Western Cape, and assumes that HIV-positive children spend 10.8 days in hospital over their short lives being treated for opportunistic infections. This results in a total cost to the health sector (for the 74 HIV-positive children resulting from 1,000 pregnancies) of R980,700.

Now let us turn to the costing of an MTCTP programme. The first component of any such programme is voluntary counselling and testing (VCT). Lines 7 to 21 of the appendix provide a costing exercise for VCT for 1,000 women. This includes provision for the costs of management, administration, HIV tests (Rapid tests and confirmatory tests) and pre- and post-test counselling. Following HIV Management Services (1998) it is assumed that after pre-test counselling, 91.5% will agree to an HIV test. Of those who test positive, it is assumed that 92.5% (i.e. 207 women) will agree to a short course of antiretroviral therapy in order to help prevent the transmission of HIV to their babies.

At this point, policy makers are faced with a choice concerning the treatment regime to provide. The following antiretroviral intervention regimes are considered:

1 A short-course AZT 'Thai' regimen (300 mg of Zidovudine every 12 hours from 36 weeks into the pregnancy and 300 mg every 3 hours

during labour). This intervention reduces mother-to-child transmission from 30% to 19%.

2 The HIVNET012 Nevirapine regimen (200 mg of Nevirapine during labour, and 2 mg per kg for the baby). This intervention reduces mother-to-child transmission from 30% to 20%.

The HIVNET012 study (based in Uganda) was subsequently mired in controversy after the US Food and Drug Administration refused to register Nevirapine as a single-dose indication for MTCTP because of administrative problems experienced during the study. An exhaustive review by the National Institutes of Health in the United States concluded that these problems had no bearing on the results, and hence recommended that Nevirapine be regarded as safe for MTCTP purposes. The Medicines Control Council of South Africa, however, decided in July 2003 to question the Ugandan study – thus threatening the registration of Nevirapine for this purpose. This move (which in the end left the status quo unchanged) was surprising, given that over 80,000 single doses of Nevirapine had been used for MTCTP purposes since the Ugandan study, resulting in the reduction of HIV transmission to between 10 and 12% (McIntyre 2003). There is no question that Nevirapine has been scientifically shown to be effective, although problems have been raised about drug resistance following a single-dose Nevirapine intervention (ibid.).

The AZT and Nevirapine treatment regimes can be implemented as such, or can be supplemented with six months of formula milk (to reduce the chances of transmitting HIV to the baby via breastfeeding). Table 3.1 summarises the results of the costing exercise for the two interventions, assuming the mothers breastfeed their babies. The AZT regimen prevents more HIV infections than the Nevirapine regimen, but it costs more – both in total, and when expressed as a cost per child saved.

Note that both the MTCTP interventions reduce, but do not eliminate, the transmission of HIV to babies. Some children still contract HIV from their mothers. These children will suffer from AIDS-related opportunistic infections during their short lives, and will be taken to public clinics and hospitals for treatment, thus costing the state money. These costs need to be added to the total health costs associated with the MTCTP programme – so as to get a full (undiscounted) picture of the burden borne by the health sector.[4] When these total costs are divided by the number of children saved from HIV-infection (to get total health costs per child saved), we see that the AZT regimen is now more cost-effective than the

Nevirapine regimen. This is because the costs of treating the opportunistic infections of those children born HIV-positive, despite the programme, tips the balance in favour of the intervention that saves the most lives (i.e. AZT).

Table 3.1 *The 'cost-effectiveness' of reducing* MTCTP *in South Africa: summary statistics for a breastfeeding population*

Assume 1,000 pregnant women, of whom 24.5% will be HIV-positive. Of these 245 women, 30% will transmit the virus to their babies, i.e. 74 babies will be infected with HIV from their mothers.	Nevirapine (HIVNET012)	AZT ('Thai' regimen)
Number of children saved as a result of an MTCTP programme for 1,000 pregnant women	20.7	22.8
Cost of the MTCTP programme per child saved (i.e. voluntary counselling and testing and a short-course of antiretroviral medication)	R3,800	R5,800
Total health costs of the MTCTP programme plus the costs of treating the opportunistic infections of HIV-positive children	R783,300	R809,300
Total health costs per child saved	R37,800	R35,500
Cost savings for the government of the MTCTP programme (i.e. total health costs without the MTCTP programme minus total health costs with the MTCTP programme)	R197,400	R171,300

Source: Appendix

If this total cost is compared with the cost of not intervening at all (i.e. R980,700), we see that it *saves* the government money to introduce MTCTP. Total health costs under an MTCTP programme (i.e. cost of MTCTP and the costs of caring for all HIV-positive children) are about R171,000 less than would be the case in the absence of an MTCTP programme (i.e. caring for all the HIV-positive children if no MTCTP programme was in place). Cost savings are higher (R197,400) for the Nevirapine regimen but, as noted above, that intervention saves fewer lives and costs more per life saved. As shown in the appendix, the government still saves money (with both programmes) if we assume that the costs of caring for HIV-positive children are reduced by 25%, and if the costs associated with the MTCTP programme are simultaneously 25% higher than expected. The results, in other words, are robust.

What policy implications can we draw from this? Assuming for the moment that these are the only two MTCTP interventions available, the government would have to decide whether to adopt the programme that saves the most lives but saves less money – or to adopt the programme that saves the most money. This is ultimately a matter of social choice. However, given that government expenditure is not normally envisaged as having the goal of saving the government money, it is likely that the favoured policy would be to save the most lives. This means favouring the AZT intervention. Potential problems relating to drug resistance from a single dose of Nevirapine (McIntyre 2003) may also tip the balance in favour of an AZT intervention.

Introducing substitute feeding

Now let us consider two further intervention options, i.e. adding substitute formula to both programmes in order to prevent the transmission of HIV to the baby during breastfeeding. There is a large body of research showing that providing infant formula to HIV-positive mothers substantially reduces the risk of mother-to-child transmission of HIV (see summary by Farley *et al.* 2000). But it is important to recognise that switching from breastfeeding to formula feeding also imposes new risks for the child – albeit from a different source. If mothers do not prepare the formula correctly, or use contaminated water, then there is a risk that the child could die from diarrhoea or respiratory diseases (Kuhn 2002a). This risk is highest in resource-poor settings where the underlying infant mortality rate is already high (Kahn *et al.* 2002; Kuhn 2002a; Kuhn and Stein 1997).

Whether the non-HIV mortality associated with substitute feeding exceeds the risk of HIV-mortality is ultimately an empirical question. Kahn *et al.* (2002) recently investigated the relative risks of different feeding strategies in urban and rural areas in four developing countries: South Africa, Tanzania, Thailand and Brazil. They found that 'the optimal feeding strategy in seven settings (all but rural Brazil) is formula feeding' (2002: 208). In the case of rural Brazil, these results were in large part a function of low reported rates of HIV transmission through breast milk (an unusual result) and high non-HIV mortality.

Judging from Kahn *et al.*'s results for South Africa, the risks of HIV-infection outweigh the risks of non-HIV-related mortality. However, this finding may not hold in very poor areas – especially in places where non-contaminated water is difficult to obtain. Under such conditions, policy makers may choose to recommend a breastfeeding strategy[5] rather than include substitute feeding as part of an intervention to reduce mother-to-child transmission. But this decision should not be taken lightly – especially given the fact that the risk of infant deaths associated with the use of substitute feeding can be substantially reduced through improved counselling about the proper preparation of formula milk and the import-ance of boiling (or otherwise sterilising) water (Forsyth and Nattrass 2002). Those who are concerned about the risks associated with substitute feeding stress the need for counsellors to 'advise mothers to understand the risks and benefits of breastfeeding and formula feeding so that they can make an informed choice. Women who choose to breastfeed can be assisted to make breastfeeding safer' (Karim *et al.* 2002: 992). However, just as counselling can advise women how to improve breastfeeding tech-niques (see Kuhn 2002a), it is equally important that counselling should also include instruction on how to avoid the risks associated with formula feeding. There are serious ethical problems with any approach that simply *assumes* that a woman from a poor area is not capable of feeding her baby properly with substitute formula and hence, for this reason, has to follow a less than optimal feeding regimen for her child. Instead, greater efforts should be made to empower women from these areas to better protect their children from both HIV-related and non-HIV mortality. Furthermore, in order to provide women with a real choice between breastfeeding and formula feeding, it is necessary for the government to provide free formula milk for indigent mothers. Otherwise, it will only be those well-off enough to purchase it themselves who will be in a position to exercise effective choice (Khoza 2002).

In the analysis that follows, it is assumed that the risk of non-HIV-related infant mortality doubles for those babies who are fed on formula milk. This is almost certainly an overestimate of the average impact in terms of additional child mortality – especially given the fact that the intervention includes counselling, and hence women will be advised on the appro-priate use of formula feeding. Table 3.2 provides summary statistics for the costing exercise for the AZT and Nevirapine regimens, but this time includ-ing six months of formula milk. More detail on the calculation is provided in the appendix. As can be seen from Tables 3.1 and 3.2, MTCTP program-mes are likely to save more lives when they include substitute feeding, than they would if the mother breastfeeds. And, while the cost of the inter-vention per child saved is higher in the substitute-feeding scenario, the

Table 3.2 *The 'cost-effectiveness' of reducing MTCTP in South Africa: summary statistics for interventions including formula feeding (rather than breastfeeding)*

Assume 1,000 pregnant women, of whom 24.5% will be HIV-positive. Of these 245 women, 30% will transmit the virus to their babies, i.e. 74 babies will be infected with HIV from their mothers.	Nevirapine (HIVNET012) with substitute feeding	AZT ('Thai' regimen) with substitute feeding
Number of lives saved as a result of the MTCTP programme for 1,000 pregnant women (i.e. the number saved from HIV infection minus the extra deaths among HIV-negative children resulting from substitute feeding)	30.2	32.1
Cost of the MTCTP programme per child saved (i.e. voluntary counselling and testing and providing antiretroviral treatment to HIV-positive women, and six months of formula milk)	R6,000	R7,300
Total health costs of the MTCTP programme plus the costs of treating the opportunistic infections of HIV-positive children	R661,500	R688,900
Total health costs per child saved	R21,900	R21,400
Cost savings for the government of the MTCTP programme (i.e. total health costs without the MTCTP programme minus total health costs with the MTCTP programme)	R319,200	R291,800

Source: Appendix

total health cost per child saved is lower. In other words, the provision of six months of infant formula results in a higher cost of the intervention, but because it saves more children from HIV infection, there are less HIV-related opportunistic infections to treat, and hence lower total health costs overall.

There are, of course, a host of potential obstacles to the use of substitute feeding that extend beyond the difficulties of preparing the infant formula correctly. These include social pressures to breastfeed and pressures from health care professionals who were trained to follow the 'breast-is-best' approach and find it difficult to shift their attitudes with regard to HIV-positive women. The World Health Organisation guidelines recommend that women be counselled about the benefits of substitute feeding and be allowed to make an informed choice that best suits their circumstances (Fowler and Newell 2000). Similar guidelines have been posted on the South African department of health website (Evian 2000). This is undoubtedly the best route forward – as long as counsellors are properly trained, and as long as women are indeed given a real choice. Mothers should be given the choice rather than having decisions made on their behalf by policy makers looking at aggregated statistics such as background infant mortality rates.

So far, the cost discussion has been presented in terms of 1,000 pregnancies. If we extend the analysis to include actual pregnancies in South Africa each year, then it can be shown that an AZT plus formula feeding regime could save about 45,000 children each year, at a direct cost of 1.6% of the health budget (mid-point estimates from Skordis and Nattrass 2002). This is broadly in line with other South African studies showing that MTCTP programmes would cost less than 3% of the health budget (see overview in Geffen 2000). Once the costs of *not* intervening (i.e. about R856 million a year) are included in the calculation, then it appears that the government is wasting about 1% of the health budget by not introducing MTCTP. This destroys the argument that South Africa cannot afford MTCTP.

But will the state actually treat the HIV-positive children for opportunistic infections?

There is a very obvious challenge to the case presented here: what if the government decides not to treat the HIV-positive children for opportunistic infections? If this happens, then the cost of not introducing MTCTP falls dramatically. Rather than treating the opportunistic infections of HIV-positive children, hospitals could be instructed to send the children home to die. Under such circumstances, the government would probably save money by not introducing MTCTP.

One answer to this would be to point out that such a policy would probably be unconstitutional. However, this sidesteps the important fact that hospitals make decisions about who to treat and who not to treat all the time. Medical practitioners in South Africa operate in a resource-constrained environment and although the situation is not as dire as the Crimean War scenario sketched in Chapter 2, medics still have to make hard choices about how to allocate resources. HIV-positive children who are terminally ill and have a limited chance of recovering from opportunistic infections are thus unlikely to receive priority treatment.

It has been reported that the paediatric ward at Dora Nginza Hospital outside Port Elizabeth tries to restrict each HIV-positive child to only one hospital admission during its life.[6] These children continue to be treated for opportunistic infections, but all subsequent care has to be clinic- and home-based. Baragwanath Hospital has also reported a downward trend in the number of days in hospital for each HIV-positive child (from 13 in 1992 to 9 in 1996 (Steinberg *et al.* 2000: 317). If this is a typical pattern, then the assumption made above that each HIV-positive child spends on average 10.8 days in hospital is probably too high.

Would a generalised Dora Nginza approach to treating the opportunistic infections of HIV-positive children reverse the conclusion that it costs the government more not to introduce MTCTP than it would to introduce it? The answer depends on the level of care accorded to HIV-positive children. Obviously, if they are denied *all* treatment the conclusion would indeed be reversed, and it would pay the government not to introduce MTCTP. But it does not take much medical care before the calculation shifts back in favour of MTCTP. For example, the appendix includes a 'limited treatment' scenario in which HIV-positive children get one hospital visit, are tested for HIV (and the mother is counselled), and are limited to nine clinic visits (costed at one quarter the cost of a hospital visit) and given R1,000 worth of medicine for home-based care over their lives.

This is a reasonable approximation of the Dora Nginza strategy. The modelling results indicate that the government still saves money, under this scenario, but it is substantially less than is the case for the best-estimate projections (see Table 3.3 and the appendix). Notice that the total health costs per child saved through MTCTP is lower in this scenario than it is for the earlier exercises. This is simply because it costs the government less to treat those children who become HIV-positive despite the intervention (because these unfortunate children would be subject to the limited treatment rule too).

Another possible objection to the costing exercises presented so far is to argue that many children (especially those in rural areas or living in poor households with limited budgets for transport) will never reach the health system, and therefore will not cost the health sector anything. Many children who are born HIV-positive simply live and die untreated. In order to model the impact of limited access to the health sector, the appendix includes the result of another costing exercise in which it is assumed that of the 1,000 pregnant women, only two thirds are in a position to take advantage of the health system, either for themselves or their children.[7] The results indicate that the numbers of children saved is lower (because fewer women participate in MTCTP) but the total health costs per child saved is also lower than the other costing exercises because fewer HIV-positive children are being treated for opportunistic infections, and because fewer women are making use of the MTCTP programme.

Table 3.3 *The Nevirapine (HIVNET012) regimen with formula feeding, assuming the 'limited treatment' and 'limited access' cost estimates*

	Limited treatment*	Limited access**
Number of lives saved as a result of the MTCTP programme (i.e. the number saved from HIV infection minus the extra deaths among HIV-negative children resulting from substitute feeding)	30.2	20.2
Cost of the MTCTP programme per child saved (i.e. voluntary counselling and testing and providing antiretroviral treatment to HIV-positive women, and six months of formula milk)	R6,000	R6,000
Total health costs of the MTCTP programme plus the costs of treating the opportunistic infections of HIV-positive children	R396,500	R220,300
Total health costs per child saved	R13,100	R10,900
Cost savings for the government of the MTCTP programme (i.e. total health costs without the MTCTP programme minus total health costs with the MTCTP programme)	R44,200	R74,900

Source: Appendix

* The limited treatment scenario assumes that HIV-positive children get one hospital visit, are tested for HIV (and the mother is counselled), and are limited to nine clinic visits (costed at one quarter the cost of a hospital visit) and are provided with R1,000 worth of medicine for home-based care.
** The limited access estimate assumes that one third of the 1,000 women do not have access to hospitals or clinics – they therefore do not parti- cipate in the programme and are not able to take their sick HIV-positive children to medical facilities for treatment of opportunistic infections. It also assumes limited treatment (as in the point above).

If one assumes that *no* HIV-positive children are ever treated for opportunistic infections, then of course the results of the costing exercises will be reversed. However, if one assumes that some limited treatment is available (as assumed above) then it will save the government money to introduce an MTCTP programme. The conclusion that 'it costs the state more to treat HIV-positive children than it does to save them from HIV' is not simply a statement about empirical reality (although it approximates it in important respects). Instead, it is probably best considered as a conditional conclusion that reads: 'unless the government has decided not to treat HIV-positive children for opportunistic infections, paediatric costs will exceed the costs of MTCTP'. The not-so-subtle charge against government officials who argue that MTCTP is 'unaffordable' becomes: 'either you have not done your economic calculus properly, or you have decided not to treat the HIV-positive children – which is it?'

What about orphans?

Before turning to the government's response to this question, it is worth considering one further objection to the costing exercise presented here – that it does not take into account the costs of orphans. This objection was made by the late presidential spokesperson Parks Mankahlana. When asked why the government was not introducing MTCTP, he replied:

That mother is going to die and that HIV-negative child will be an orphan. That child must be brought up, who is going to bring that child up? It's the state, the state. That's resources you see (quoted in the American Magazine *Science*, and reported in the electronic *Mail and Guardian*, 22 December 2000).

Remarks such as these give the unfortunate impression that the South African government was deliberately trying to reduce the number of AIDS orphans by ensuring that as many of them as possible contracted HIV. Such arguments are reminiscent of the economically rational, but socially unacceptable, policies outlined in Chapter 1. No wonder, then, that the *Mail and Guardian* observed in an editorial that the government 'should not be surprised to hear charges of genocide directed against it' (21 July 2000).

But let us pause for a moment and consider Mankahlana's economic argument seriously. Would the government save money by increasing the numbers of HIV-positive orphans (as opposed to reducing the numbers through an MTCTP programme)? For this to happen, several (implausible) conditions must hold. First, it must be the case that HIV-positive children die quickly and without imposing any costs on the government. The fact that paediatric wards in hospitals are flooded with HIV-positive children,[8] together with evidence that many HIV-positive children reach school-going age, quickly puts paid to that assumption.

Second, it must be the case that increasing the number of HIV-positive children relative to HIV-negative children will result in fewer children being abandoned into state care. The vast majority of orphans, both HIV-positive and HIV-negative, are cared for by extended families (Gow and Desmond 2002). As the burden imposed by AIDS gets ever greater for households, it is likely that more children will be abandoned as extended families reach a point at which they can no longer support the children. But consider for a moment which children are likely to be abandoned first: the HIV-positive, or the HIV-negative? Given that the burden of care is so much greater for HIV-positive children, and given that 'investing' in HIV-positive children is unlikely ever to yield a return in terms of future earnings, it stands to reason that HIV-positive children are likely to be abandoned first. The growing numbers of abandoned HIV-positive children in state-funded and private-funded hospices and shelters is testimony to this kind of decision making. It is thus possible that *more* children will be abandoned into state care if the government failed to introduce MTCTP programmes than would be the case if they did.

If so, then what on the face of it seemed to be an economically rational argument (albeit unpalatable) from Parks Mankahlana, is in fact not economically rational after all. Indeed, if one pauses to consider *other* government expenditure on children, the case for not introducing MTCTP programmes becomes incoherent. Governments invest in children in many ways, the most obvious being in the provision of education and child support grants. The implicit expectation of such policies is that once the children grow up, they will be able to compensate society for the earlier investment by becoming productive, tax-paying adults. In terms of this economic understanding of the social contract to educate and provide for children, it makes no sense whatsoever to increase the numbers of children with a terminal illness (as implied by Mankahlana). This is particularly the case with regard to the child support grant, which provides income to indigent care-givers of children up to the age of fourteen. For HIV-negative children, this expenditure can be seen as a form of investment. For HIV-positive children, it can be regarded only as an unrecoverable form of consumption spending.

3.3 The government's response: a moral economy of triage?

An earlier version of the net-cost calculations summarised in Tables 3.1 and 3.2 was presented as part of an expert affidavit in support of TAC's case against the government (Nattrass 2001a). It argued (as above) that there was no basis for the government's claim that a national MTCTP programme is unaffordable. The director general of health, Dr Ayanda Ntsaluba, wrote the main replying affidavit on the part of the government, and addressed this argument in some detail.[9]

The issue of resource availability

One of the responses which Ntsaluba made to Nattrass (2001a) was that the argument failed to consider the 'organisational and logistic challenges which must be overcome *en route*' (par. 227.2.4). This criticism has validity, especially with regard to the poorer provinces, where health services (particularly in rural areas) are under-resourced and mismanaged. In such areas it would take more resources in the short-term to initiate MTCTP than included in my estimates (see appendix). However, even if we were to *triple* the costs of the voluntary counselling and testing estimate, the results (including those for the sensitivity analysis) are still cost-saving for the government for all MTCTP scenarios.

This, however, was not the main criticism. The centrepiece of Ntsaluba's economic argument was that the introduction of MTCTP would have a negative effect on the public sector because of the extra strain it would place on resources: 'should the existing staff be required to take on, for example, counselling duties, this is likely to have a huge impact on the quality and quantity of the other services which are provided in the public sector' (par. 23.4). Anticipating the obvious retort (that more counsellors should be hired), he went on to argue that it is 'not easy simply to decide to employ more people within the current budgets as this displaces funds from other areas such as medicines and equipment' (par. 23.5). Several pages further on, he defended the failure of provincial governments to implement MTCTP by saying that they were doing everything they could under the 'difficult circumstances' they found themselves in, and that they were 'forced to make difficult and painful choices' given the 'numerous competing and equally important demands on the limited resources under their control' (par. 30.1).

Statements such as these are evocative of the Crimean War field hospital: too many people needing treatment, but too few resources. It is a moral economy of triage: embattled health ministers are doing the best they can under difficult circumstances, they have to make hard choices, and MTCTP just doesn't make the cut-off point. Like those badly wounded soldiers requiring too many resources in relation to their chances of recovery, the MTCTP programme is portrayed as having to die alone outside.

What is wrong with this picture? Chapter 2 argued that the moral economy of triage is only reasonable in extreme situations where two conditions exist: (1) resources are absolutely constrained, and (2) the allocation of resources is a zero-sum game. Taking the second point first, the central argument made in this chapter is that the allocation of resources is *not* a zero-sum game. Money spent to prevent HIV infections means less future expenditure on AIDS-related opportunistic infections. The analogy of the field hospital no longer holds. Rather than looking myopically at individual cases needing immediate treatment, policy makers should rather be thinking about the flow of medical cases into hospitals over time. As argued in Section 3.2, MTCTP programmes more than pay for themselves by reducing the flow of AIDS-related paediatric cases to government health facilities. The budget process (which is currently focussed on short-term budget cycles) needs to be revised in order to accommodate such considerations.[10]

Now consider point 1. Are health resources absolutely constrained? According to the affidavits by Ntsaluba and the provincial MECs,[11] this is the case. Asking health personnel to counsel women as part of an MTCTP programme means that they will have less time to help other patients – and if we hire more counsellors, this means there will be less medicine and equipment. While appearing to concede the point about cost-effectiveness over time, Ntsaluba highlights the constraints that exist on start-up costs:

[W]hat is cost-effective may not be affordable in the short-term. The argument that because it is cost-effective, it can immediately be done is simplistic. Clearly, additional resources will be needed in the short-term. In the longer term of course, this may be compensated by the costs of care averted, but this does not deal with the immediate problems (par. 127.3).

In other words, we are back in the Crimean field hospital with limited supplies and no hope of replenishing them while the fighting lasts. This, however, is also an incorrect analogy. The health budget, like any other budget, is limited by available resources. But the size of each budget within this resource envelope is a product of social choice. It is quite possible that after having been presented with the argument in favour of allocating resources to MTCTP, most people would accept an initial increase in the size of the health budget to accommodate it. After all, the prospect of saving the lives of ('innocent') babies is likely to have wide-spread appeal – especially if the public understands that the programme will pay for itself in the short- to medium-term (by averting health expenditure on AIDS-sick children). Appealing to the limited resources in the health sector as a reason for inaction begs the very question of social choice. We can, in other words, choose to send more supplies to the field hospital. Given that this initial investment will more than pay for itself (in terms of later savings to the health sector), opting for such a route forward is both reasonable/moral and economically rational.

What has been happening to health expenditure on AIDS?

What is South Africa currently spending on AIDS? Unfortunately it is impossible to place an exact figure on AIDS-related government expend-iture because it occurs in a range of budgets (education, health, welfare) and entails a host of hidden costs such as treating opportunistic infections and personnel costs pertaining to HIV infection among government employees. The situation is complicated further by the fact that revenues are collected centrally and allocated to provinces according to the 'equit-able share' formula. Apart from a few conditional grants from national to provincial governments (which have to be used for the purposes they were earmarked for), provincial governments can decide how to allocate their resources between competing objectives. Thus even if the national government allocates more money to provinces for AIDS (as was the case in the 2003/4 budget), it has 'no legal means of making sure that provinces do spend the money on HIV/AIDS treatment strategies as intended' (Hickey 2002: 1271).

Government budgetary allocations are presented over a 'medium-term expenditure framework' (MTEF). The national treasury has introduced a specific budget item earmarked for fighting AIDS in the health sector – the 'Enhanced Response to HIV/AIDS Strategy'. It is effected by increases in the equitable share allocation of revenue to provincial governments and is over and above three conditional AIDS-related grants to the departments of health, education and social development. In the first phase of the 'Enhanced Response' budgetary allocation, spending was envisaged to rise from R345 million in 2001/2 to over R1 billion in 2002/3 to R1.8 billion in 2004/5. This included expenditure for basic preventive interventions such as life-skills training, condom provision, voluntary counselling and testing, MTCTP, support for the South African AIDS Vaccine Initiative, co-funding the LoveLife Programme and the treatment of sexually transmitted infections.[12] It also provided funding to strengthen programme management at provincial level. In the 2003/4 budget, a further R3.3 billion was made available for possible addition to provincial allocations to be spent on the Enhanced Response to HIV/AIDS Strategy over the MTEF (Treasury 2003a: 87–8). According to the national treasury: 'In addition to strengthening preventive programmes and supporting full rollout of the mother-to-child and post-exposure programmes, the 2003 Budget provides for a substantial boost to care and treatment programmes' (ibid. 88).

In other words, it would appear that at least in the eyes of the national treasury sufficient funds have now been allocated for a 'full rollout' of MTCTP programmes. This was achieved without an increase in the share of health spending in total consolidated government expenditure. If this is the case, then it indicates that, in contrast to the protestations of the various provincial ministers of health in their affidavits to the constitutional court, the additional resources required in the short term were not excessive.

However, as the Financial and Fiscal Commission (FFC) has recently warned:

The fact that the HIV/AIDS increment to the provincial equitable share is not ring-fenced in any way raises concerns that the allocation may not be used to cover the direct costs of HIV/AIDS ... Investigations carried out by the FFC in KwaZulu-Natal and the Eastern Cape could not find any indication that allocations to any function affected by HIV/AIDS directly received this money (quoted in the *Cape Times*, 16 May 2003).

Table 3.4 provides some data for health spending since 1999, and its projection forward according to the MTEF. There are two striking features of Table 3.4 with regard to health. Firstly, the vast bulk of South Africa's health spending takes place through provincial budgets; and secondly, the share of total spending on health fell between 1999 and 2002 and is projected to fall further (as a share of both national and provincial budgets).

Note that the fall in expenditure on health in the provinces in 1999/2000 occurred at a time when the provinces had a surplus of revenue over expenditure. This suggests that it was not as a result of a shortage of financial resources that the provinces experienced slow growth in real health expenditure. According to the national treasury: 'While substantial proportions of the surpluses were planned for repayment of debts, part of the surpluses reflects the lack of capacity to spend' (2003b: 22).

While provinces most certainly experience skills shortages and the poorer provinces have demonstrably weak administrations, this 'lack of capacity to spend' cannot be placed solely at the door of objective constraints. The failure to spend available resources must also be laid, in part, at the door of a political failure to act. In some provinces, this failure to act

Table 3.4 *Trends in government expenditure*

	Actual spending		Estimated actual		Medium-term estimates		
	1999/0	2000/1	2001/2	2002/3	2003/4	2004/5	2005/6
Real growth in total provincial spending	−2.4%	2.4%	3.2%	10.6%	7.4%	4.2%	5.5%
Real growth in provincial health spending	−2.1%	1.7%	5.7%	5.1%	4.5%	3.3%	3.3%
Provincial surpluses (+) and deficits (−) (Rmillion)	3,527	3,347	3,777	−2,327	−1,127	−99	−1,080
Shares in total provincial spending							
Education	39.8%	39.1%	38.3%	36.7%	35.6%	35.1%	34.0%
Health	24.1%	23.9%	24.3%	22.9%	22.3%	22.1%	21.6%
Social development	19.4%	18.9%	19.4%	18.8%	22.9%	24.4%	25.8%
% of consolidated national and provincial expenditure on health	14.3%	14.3%	14.0%	13.3%	13.1%	13.1%	13.0%
Total government spending as % of GDP	27.2%	26.7%	27.0%	27.7%	28.5%	28.3%	28.3%
Total tax revenue as % of GDP	24.2%	23.6%	24.6%	24.6%	24.7%	24.6%	24.6%

Source: Treasury (2003b: 15, 16); Treasury (2003a: 76, 210–11); South African Reserve Bank

is both a product of poor commitment to policy implementation and financial mismanagement. The Eastern Cape is the prime example of this. In the 2000/1 financial year, the Eastern Cape allocated R33 million to HIV/AIDS projects which were, according to the MEC for health, 'ready to be rolled out throughout the Province from the 1st April' (quoted in Allan and Vitsha 2001: 1). However, almost none of this money was spent. When the Auditor-General's office examined the financial statements for the department of health, it drew attention to the failure as a 'matter of emphasis':

HIV/AIDS related projects are regarded as high priority spending by the department, the province and the country as a whole, yet the department failed to utilise the money. The amount unspent had not been 'rolled forward' to the new financial year by the National Treasury and was therefore lost to the province (Auditor-General's report, cited in Allan and Vitsha 2001: 2).

The fact that none of this money was spent – and that no effort had been made to roll-over the funds to the following year – points to an extraordinary failure of leadership at all ministerial levels. It cannot simply be placed at the door of 'implementation challenges' or 'legacies of the past' (although the lack of control by national decision makers over the spending decisions of provinces is a legacy of South Africa's negotiated political settlement). According to a report by Anso Thom in the *Mail and Guardian* (27 June 2003 to 3 July 2003), South Africa's MTCTP programme, with the exception of Gauteng, KwaZulu-Natal and the Western Cape, is a 'shambles'. Outside of these provinces, very few pregnant women are being reached, national staff fail to attend key meetings, provincial posts have not been filled for over a year, and there is a chaotic approach to planning. The report states:

There are charges that it is not in the interests of some denialist politicians for the MTCTP programme to succeed, as this is the first step towards a state-sponsored anti-retroviral treatment plan. Getting the drugs to the hospitals and clinics is the easy part. Ensuring that there is the political will for effective implementation on the part of premiers and their provincial ministers is an entirely different matter. (ibid.)

This is not, of course, to downplay the challenges of building a better health system. As can be seen from the selected data in Table 3.5, there are significant inequalities in health care provision between the provinces.

Table 3.5 *Selected provincial public health data*

	Expenditure per capita 2002/3	% children fully immunised at 1 year	Antenatal coverage rate (% having at least one visit) 2002	Antenatal visits per antenatal attender 2002	Hospital beds per 1,000 public users	Hospital admissions per 1,000 uninsured population (2001/2)	Bed occupancy in regional hospitals
Eastern Cape	668	60.0%	77.0%	3.3	2.8	70.1	48%
Free State	969	82.0%	100.0%	4.3	2.2	95.9	66%
Gauteng	1,580	64.0%	78.0%	3.8	3.5	151.8	70%
KwaZulu-Natal	939	77.0%	89.0%	4.0	3.5	127.7	69%
Limpopo	586	67.0%	82.0%	3.9	2.1	71.5	62%
Mpuma-langa	635	80.0%	100.0%	3.7	1.6	75.3	63%
Northern Cape	876	65.0%	63.0%	4.0	2.4	194.3	95%
North West	628	71.0%	82.0%	4.2	1.8	66.9	74%
Western Cape	1,261	65.0%	79.0%	4.7	3.4	154.7	88%
Total	911	70.0%	79.0%	3.9	2.8	104.9*	67%

Source: National treasury 2003b: 77, 86, 89, 90. * Total admissions = 3,761,557

The 'equitable share' allocation of government revenue to provinces takes into account the greater needs of poorer provinces and thus it is to be expected that these inequalities will narrow over time. However, given the relatively slow overall projected increase in health expenditure, such inequalities are likely to remain significant over the foreseeable future. Specific attention must thus be paid to the needs and capabilities of poorer provinces when it comes to rolling out MTCTP programmes. In areas where the health system is badly managed at local and provincial level (as appears to be the case in the Eastern Cape), the onus is on the national government to provide targeted managerial and financial support.

To end this discussion on a slightly optimistic note, it is encouraging to see that antenatal coverage is reasonably high in South Africa. Most women visit a health care facility at least once during their pregnancy – with an average of almost four visits per antenatal attender. According to data from the demographic and health survey, 83% of births are attended by a medically trained person (Booysen 2002a: 399). Taken together, this suggests that the network of clinics is sufficiently dense that pregnant women are able to make use of them – and that they form a basis upon which to develop a national MTCTP programme. The challenge is thus to upgrade the services provided at the clinics and medical facilities to provide for MTCTP. The fact that provincial underspending on conditional grants has declined (Hickey and Ndlovu 2003: 14) is perhaps grounds for cautious optimism about provincial capacity to deliver on health programmes.[13]

According to a report compiled in early 2002 by the Health Systems Trust on the government's eighteen pilot MTCTP sites, some provinces are in a better position than others to introduce MTCTP programmes (and thus should move at different speeds). The report concludes that 'with political and senior management commitment at both national and provincial level, it should be possible for all provinces to begin implementing MTCTP services in some new sites by the middle of 2002' (cited in TAC 2002). Given the reputation that the Health Systems Trust has developed for continually pointing to implementation problems when AIDS-implementation policies are proposed,[14] this conclusion is particularly welcome.

3.4 How many children could be saved from HIV infection?

So far the discussion has been conducted solely in terms of costs to the health sector. Neither the costs to parents of having terminally ill children to care for, nor the value of a human life have been considered. This is because the agenda for the analysis was set by the government's long-standing claim that it could 'not afford' to implement an MTCTP programme. The analysis thus, inevitably, focussed on the direct costs and costs averted for the public health sector rather than society at large.

In this concluding part of the chapter it is worth taking a step back and considering the larger picture. If South Africa implemented a full roll-out of MTCTP, how many children could be saved? To answer this, it is helpful to consult South Africa's leading demographic model: ASSA2000. This model estimates the impact of AIDS on the South African population. It uses data from the 1998–2000 antenatal clinic surveys, the 1998 South

African demographic and health survey and best estimates of population and mortality.[15] The model includes various parameters of heterosexual behaviour (such as the probability that a partner comes from a particular risk group, the number of sexual partners per annum, the age of the partner, and the probability that a condom is used during intercourse). These parameters have been 'calibrated' (i.e. adjusted) so that the model's results match the results of the annual antenatal clinic surveys both in terms of overall level and age. This can be seen in Figure 3.1, which plots actual antenatal survey data (by age) and projected HIV prevalence, for both the total population and antenatal clinic attendees. The ASSA2000 model predicts that HIV prevalence in the South African population will peak at 14.6% in 2005, whereas the projected prevalence levels for young women attending antenatal clinics will reach 35% by 2020.

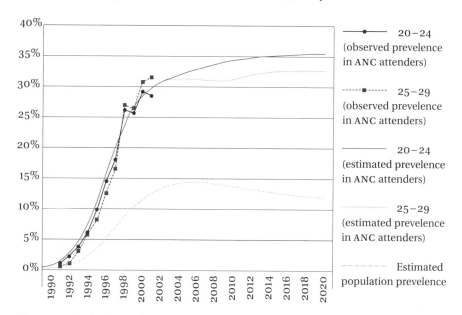

Figure 3.1 *Projections of HIV prevalence from the ASSA2000 demographic model and the antenatal clinic survey (1990–2020)*

According to the model, HIV prevalence in South Africa was 13.2% in 2001. This is higher than that measured by the 2001 national household survey (Shisana and Simbayi 2002: 45). According to this study, total HIV-prevalence in South Africa was 11.4% (with a 95% confidence interval of 10.0% to 12.7%). However, there were serious problems of bias in this survey,[16] and hence it is likely that overall prevalence is closer to that estimated by the ASSA2000 model.

More recently an ASSA2000 Interventions Model has been developed to estimate the demographic impact of various AIDS prevention and treatment interventions.[17] This model (which is discussed more fully in Chapter 4) enables us to compare the impact of MTCTP programmes compared to a 'no interventions' scenario. The model assumes that a national voluntary counselling and testing programme is implemented, that the government implements a Nevirapine regimen for HIV-positive pregnant women, and offers women the option of six months' (free) supply of formula milk.[18] The model assumes that only 50% of women opt to use substitute feeding rather than breastfeeding. According to a *Lancet* reviewer of a costing study using the ASSA2000 Interventions Model, the assumption that only half of the women will accept formula milk is 'worrisome'. He observes that 'for the sake of South Africa's children, I sincerely hope the authors are wrong' (Decosas 2003: 1146). Decosas is clearly adding his voice to the pro-substitute feeding lobby. The import of the assumption for the ASSA2000 Interventions Model is that the output (in terms of lives saved and cost per life saved) is probably underestimated by assuming that only 50% of women take up this option.

The model assumes that the intervention is phased in over time with coverage rising from 10% in 2001 (the hypothetical start of the MTCTP intervention) to 90% in 2006. Figure 3.2 traces the number of HIV infections averted between 2001 and 2015. The number of child infections averted rises sharply for six years and then flattens out. Between 2001 and 2015, 352,800 child infections are averted by the programme. According to a costing exercise that accompanied the ASSA2000 Interventions Model, this amounts to a direct cost of R5,601 per child HIV infection averted (which is in line with the costing exercise outlined in the appendix).[19] Note that these direct costs do not include the 'savings' resulting from hospital and other medical costs averted through lower HIV infection among children. As argued in Section 3.2, if the cost calculation takes this into account, it would almost certainly be cost-saving for the government to introduce an MTCTP programme.

A striking aspect of Figure 3.2 is that it includes an estimate of adult HIV infections averted as part of the estimate of the impact of introducing MTCTP. As can be seen from the figure, the number of adult HIV infections averted rises almost to the same level (44% of the total) as that for children. Between 2001 and 2015, 279,000 adult HIV infections are averted as a result of the introduction of an MTCTP programme. This result – which at first glance may seem somewhat surprising – is a function of the assumption in the ASSA2000 Interventions Model that the voluntary counselling and testing (which accompanies an MTCTP programme) contributes to some sexual behaviour change among the women being counselled. An MTCTP programme entails pre- and post-test counselling for all women – whether they turn out to be HIV-positive or negative. Everyone thus benefits from the information and counselling that is part of this process. The ASSA2000 Interventions Model assumes that counselling encourages safer sexual behaviour (although the benefits are assumed to wear off over time). It is this increase in safer sexual behaviour among a particularly vulnerable cohort that results in the benefits of adult infections averted shown in Figure 3.2. These behavioural assumptions are discussed in more detail in Chapters 4 and 5.

The model estimates that MTCTP would save a total of 632,000 HIV infections. According to the accompanying costing exercise, this amounts to an average direct cost of R3,126 per HIV infection averted. (Note, again, that this does not include any estimate for costs averted – i.e. the 'savings'

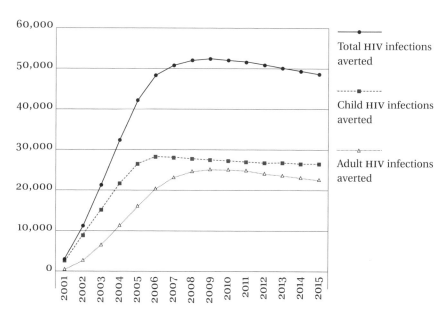

Figure 3.2 *Estimated HIV infections averted by a national MTCTP programme (ASSA2000 Interventions Model)*

to the state from having to treat fewer opportunistic infections among HIV-positive adults and children.)

Figure 3.3 considers the question of orphans. As noted in Section 3.3, concerns have been raised about the 'costs' of creating new (uninfected) orphans through an MTCTP programme. Leaving aside the ethical and practical issues that were addressed earlier, it is worth noting that these extra orphans are only a small proportion of the overall numbers of uninfected orphans that are being generated each year as a result of the AIDS pandemic. Recall that most HIV-positive pregnant women do not transmit HIV to their babies, and that not all those who participate in MTCTP programmes succeed in preventing HIV transmission to their babies. Hence, the numbers of uninfected orphans created by an MTCTP programme (relative to the numbers of uninfected orphans being created every day by the AIDS pandemic) is likely to be small. According to the ASSA2000 Interventions Model, the proportion of new uninfected orphans arising from an MTCTP programme amounts to only 8.7% of the total number of uninfected orphans born to women who died HIV-positive in 2015.

The fact that new (uninfected) orphans are being created through an

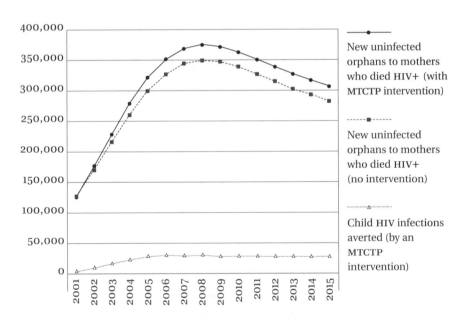

Figure 3.3 *The number of uninfected orphans of mothers who died HIV-positive with and without an MTCTP programme (ASSA2000 Interventions Model)*

MTCTP programme immediately raises the issue of saving adults. By extending the lives of HIV-positive parents, fewer children will have to grow up without their mother and/or father. One of the ethical difficulties with an MTCTP programme is precisely that it is targeted at saving the lives of infants and does not consider the treatment needs of HIV-positive parents and other adults. What would be the costs and benefits of expanding the MTCTP programme to include treatment for all who need it? Chapter 4 addresses this challenging question.

Appendix: Costing mother-to-child transmission prevention

	Best estimate	Cost sensitivity analysis		Limited treatment*	Limited access**
For every 1,000 pregnant women					
Number of HIV-positive women (24.5% × 1,000)	245	245		245	245
Number of HIV-positive babies [I] (30% × 245)	73.5	73.5		73.5	73.5
Inpatient costs for HIV-positive children [II]	980,700	735,500	⇩25%	440,600	295,200
Cost of pre-test counselling [III]	18,200	22,800	⇧25%	18,200	12,200
Cost of the Rapid tests [IV]	15,400	19,200	⇧25%	15,400	10,300
Cost of all confirmatory tests [V]	1,700	2,200	⇧25%	1,700	1,200
Post-test counselling for all HIV-negative women [VI]	2,600	3,200	⇧25%	2,600	1,700
Post-test counselling for all HIV-positive women	4,100	5,100	⇧25%	4,100	2,700
Site costs (management, phones, etc.) for all pregnant women visiting the clinic [VII]	33,000	41,300	⇧25%	33,000	22,100
Total voluntary counselling and testing (VTC) costs	74,900	93,700		74,900	50,200
The number of HIV-positive women who will accept ARV therapy [VIII]	207.4	207.4		207.4	138.9

	Best estimate	Cost sensitivity analysis		Limited treatment*	Limited access**
AZT *(Thai regimen)*					
Total cost of AZT therapy [IX]	58,100	72,600	⇧25%	58,100	38,900
Number of HIV-positive children despite the ARV programme [X]	39.4	39.4		39.4	26.4
Inpatient costs of these HIV-positive children	525,700	394,300		236,200	158,300
Number of HIV-positive children of non-participants	11.3	11.3		11.3	31.8
Inpatient costs of the HIV-positive children of non participants	150,700	113,000		67,700	0
Total health costs under Thai regimen	809,300	673,500		436,900	247,400
Number of children saved***	22.8	22.8		22.8	15.3
Total costs per child saved	35,500	29,500		19,200	16,200
Cost savings****	171,300	62,000		3,700	47,900
Cost of VCT+ARV per child saved	5,800	7,300		5,800	5,800
*Nevirapine (*HIVNET012*)*					
Total cost of ARV therapy [XI]	4,400	5,400	⇧25%	4,400	2,900
Number of HIV-positive children despite the intervention [XII]	41.5	41.5		41.5	27.8
Inpatient costs of children born HIV-positive despite MTCTP [XIII]	553,400	415,000		248,600	166,600
Inpatient costs of HIV-positive children of non-participants	150,700	113,000		67,700	0
Total health costs	783,300	627,100		395,600	219,700
Number of children saved***	20.7	20.7		20.7	13.9
Total health costs per child saved	37,800	30,200		19,100	15,800
Cost savings****	197,400	108,400		45,000	75,500
Cost of VCT+ARV per child saved	3,800	4,800		3,800	3,800

	Best estimate	Cost sensitivity analysis		Limited treatment*	Limited access**
AZT (Thai regimen) with substitute feeding (SF) for 6 months					
Total cost of AZT therapy	58,100	72,600	⇧25%	58,100	38,900
Cost of SF for 6 months XIV	103,500	129,400	⇧25%	103,500	69,400
Number of HIV-positive children despite MTCTP XV	20.7	20.7		20.7	13.9
Inpatient costs of these HIV-positive children	276,700	207,500		124,300	83,300
Inpatient costs of HIV-positive children of the non-participants	150,700	113,000		67,700	0
Number of children who die as a result of the SF XVI	10.4	13.0	⇧25%	10.4	7.0
Number of additional deaths among HIV-positive children	1.0	1.3		1.0	0.7
Number of additional deaths among HIV-negative children	9.3	11.7		9.3	6.3
Assume these children die after 3 months. Savings on SF	2,600	4,000		2,600	1,700
Medical costs of children who die as a result of SF XVII	41,500	38,900		18,600	12,500
Inpatient costs of HIV-positive babies adjusted for these early deaths	262,800	194,500		118,100	79,100
Total health costs under Thai regimen with SF	688,900	638,000		438,400	248,400
Number of children saved***	32.1	29.8		32.1	21.5
Total health costs per child saved	21,400	21,400		13,600	11,500
Cost savings****	291,800	97,500		2,300	46,900
Cost of VCT+ARV+SF per child saved	7,300	9,800		7,300	7,300

	Best estimate	Cost sensitivity analysis		Limited treatment*	Limited access**
Nevirapine regimen with substitute feeding (SF) for 6 months					
Cost of ARV therapy	4,400	5,400		4,400	2,900
Total cost of SF	103,500	129,400	⇧25%	103,500	69,400
Number of HIV-positive children despite MTCTP [XVIII]	22.8	22.8		22.8	15.3
Inpatient costs of these HIV-positive children	304,300	228,300		136,700	91,600
Inpatient costs of HIV-positive children of non-participants	150,700	113,000		67,700	0
Number of children who die as a result of SF	10.4	13.0	⇧25%	10.4	7.0
Number of additional deaths among HIV-positive children	1.1	1.4		1.1	0.8
Number of additional deaths among HIV-negative children	9.2	11.5		9.2	6.2
Assume these children die after 3 months. Savings on SF	2,600	4,000		2,600	1,700
Medical costs of children who die as a result of SF	41,500	38,900		18,600	12,500
Inpatient costs of HIV-positive babies adjusted for these early deaths	289,100	214,000		129,900	87,000
Total health costs	661,500	590,40		396,500	220,300
Number of children saved***	30.2	27.9		30.2	20.2
Total health costs per child saved	21,900	21,200		13,100	10,900
Cost savings****	319,200	145,200		44,200	74,900
Cost of VCT+ARV+SF per child saved	6,000	8,100		6,000	6,000

* The limited treatment scenario assumes that HIV-positive children get one hospital visit, are tested for HIV (and the mother is counselled), and are limited to nine clinic visits (costed at one quarter the cost of a hospital visit) and are provided with R1,000 worth of medicine for home-based care.

** The limited access estimate assumes that one third of the 1,000 women do not have access to hospitals or clinics – they therefore do not participate in the programme and are not able to take their sick HIV-positive children to medical facilities for treatment of opportunistic infections. It also assumes limited treatment (as in the point above).

*** The number of children who would be born HIV-positive in the absence of MTCTP (73.5) minus the number of HIV-positive children born to MTCTP participants and non-participants.

**** Total costs to the health sector in the absence of MTCTP minus total health costs with MTCTP.

NB: All cost estimates are in 2001 prices, and there is no discounting for costs incurred in the future. Figures do not add up exactly because of rounding errors.

I As reported in the West African pooled analysis, cited by Farley *et al.* (2000).

II Hospital costs per HIV+ child assumes that the paediatric costs of a child with AIDS is equal to 10.8 days in hospital in a high-cost hospital bed (R13,342.70 per night). No additional costing is included for medicines. This proxy for the paediatric costs of HIV/AIDS is 15% lower than the average data for paediatric costs reported in Tanzania, Zaïre and Thailand (reported in Marseille *et al.* 1999).

III Information obtained from the Western Cape HIV/AIDS Directorate. This is based on a salary of R2,000 per month per counsellor. Each counsellor has five appointments a day for twenty-two days a month. According to the Western Cape HIV/AIDS Directorate, the national government has proposed a R500 per month stipend per lay-counsellor. Using this number would substantially lower the cost of preventing MTCT.

IV Information from the Western Cape HIV/AIDS Directorate (adjusted to take into account the cost of the nurse's time to administer the test).

V This includes the cost of the Smartcheck confirmatory test and an additional Elisa test (and needles and tubes) for the 5% of indeterminate test results. Information from the Western Cape HIV/AIDS Directorate.

VI Based on counselling costs from the Western Cape HIV/AIDS Directorate (assuming five in a group). An individual counselling session costed at the same rate as the pre-test counselling session (note III). The calculation assumes that 91.5% of women presenting at the clinic agree to be tested.

VII This includes the cost of stationery, phones, photocopies, transport, mentoring for nurses and the cost of a project manager for each site, assuming 5,000 pregnancies per year per site (information from the Western Cape HIV/AIDS Directorate).

VIII This assumes that 92.5% of HIV-positive women will accept ARV therapy for MTCTP.

IX Data from the Western Cape.

X Based on 37% effectiveness reported in the West African pooled analysis cited by Farley *et al.* (2000).

XI It is assumed that the government purchases Nevirapine at the current state-tender price. However, Boehringer Ingelheim, the manufacturers of Nevirapine, have offered to donate Nevirapine to the government.

XII Based on the 35% efficacy rate after 12 months of breastfeeding, reported in Farley *et al.* (2000).

XIII See note II.

XIV This is based on a tin of formula milk (Pelargon, costing R10.40), and a child needing eight tins a month (information supplied by the Western Cape HIV/AIDS Directorate).

XV Based on results surveyed in Farley et al. (2000).

XVI We assume that the background infant mortality rate is 50 per 1,000 and that it doubles as a result of the substitute feeding. This figure will vary from more than doubling in very poor areas, to hardly increasing at all in higher-income areas. According to Evian (2000), infant mortality in South Africa varies from 24 to 103 per 1,000, and averages at about 41 per 1,000.

XVII These hospital costs are assumed to be 30% of the costs associated with children born HIV-positive who do not die as a result of the SF.

XVIII Based on the evidence from a Kenyan study that breastfeeding increases transmission by 44%, as reported in Wood (2001).

4 Expanding an AIDS intervention to include HAART for all who need it

Chapter 3 argued that an MTCTP programme would more than pay for itself because fewer children would become HIV-positive – thus resulting in a lower overall cost to the health sector. Can a similar case be made for the provision of chronic highly active antiretroviral therapy (HAART) for those already living with AIDS? Could a HAART intervention 'pay for itself' by averting AIDS-related morbidity and by encouraging people to be tested and counselled – thereby contributing to behaviour change and lower rates of HIV transmission?

This is a much tougher question to answer because the direct costs are so high, and because the benefits are in large part dependent on the validity of the assumptions used to model the impact of the intervention. The analysis presented in this chapter integrates a detailed costing exercise with the output of the ASSA2000 Interventions Model. It draws on work presented in more detail in Geffen *et al.* (2003). This study is one of several publicly available costing studies of antiretroviral provision in South Africa (see review by Boulle *et al.* 2003 and JHTTT 2003). Although some of the input data and modelling assumptions occur in all studies, they are sufficiently different to prevent direct comparisons. The study presented here is the most detailed and produces the highest cost estimates. It can thus be regarded as the 'worst-case scenario' from a cost perspective.

The ASSA2000 Interventions Model, which is an adaptation of the ASSA2000 model, was designed to estimate the likely impact of various HIV/AIDS health policy interventions.[1] While based on similar principles governing other international AIDS policy models (e.g. Stover *et al.* 2002), the ASSA2000 Interventions Model is one of the most sophisticated models of its kind. This is partly because South African socio-economic data is relatively rich, thus enabling the modellers to construct detailed parameters relating to demographic and behavioural variables.

The ASSA2000 Interventions Model was introduced in Chapter 3 (Section 3.4) to help shed light on the question of how many children could be saved from HIV infection through an MTCTP programme. Section 4.1 discusses the costs and benefits of several HIV prevention interventions, Section 4.2 considers a national HAART treatment intervention, and Section 4.3 shows that there is an economic case for including HAART as part of a broader strategy to combat AIDS.

4.1 The impact of a limited AIDS intervention

The ASSA2000 Interventions Model models HIV-transmission in South Africa as a function of sexual behaviour. It includes various parameters of heterosexual behaviour (such as the probability that a partner comes from a particular risk group, the number of sexual partners per annum, the age of the partner, and the probability that a condom is used during intercourse). Relevant South African data was obtained from the demographic and health surveys, the antenatal clinic survey and the best available estimates regarding mortality. As discussed in Chapter 3, the various parameters have been 'calibrated' (i.e. adjusted) so that the model's estimates are consistent with the results of the annual antenatal clinic surveys.

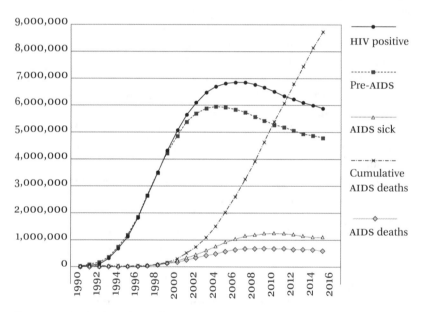

Figure 4.1 *Projections from the ASSA2000 Interventions Model of demographic trends in the absence of any AIDS prevention and treatment interventions*

The model is designed to project the number of HIV-positive people at different stages of the disease over time. It draws on several empirical studies (mostly from Africa) to estimate parameters for how fast people move from being HIV-positive but largely asymptomatic (Stages 1 and 2) to experiencing AIDS-related complexes (Stage 3) and full-blown AIDS (Stage 4).[2] As HIV-positive people are at their most infectious during the later stages of the disease, different HIV transmission probabilities are estimated for different stages of the disease.[3] This is partly counter-balanced by a factor which captures the decline in sexual activity as people progress through the different stages.[4]

Figure 4.1 traces some of the demographic projections of the ASSA2000 Interventions Model assuming no HIV/AIDS prevention or treatment interventions. As can be seen from the figure, the number of HIV-positive cases peaks in 2006, but the number of AIDS-sick individuals peaks in 2010. AIDS deaths also follow with a lag (peaking in 2009). The lag between peaks in HIV infection and in AIDS-illness and death reflects the lag between HIV-infection and the onset of illness. The cumulative increase in AIDS deaths indicates that by 2015 about 8,700,000 people will have died of AIDS. This rises to 14,400,000 in 2025. Life expectancy falls from 62 years of age in 2001 to 49 in 2025.

The model explores the impact of four AIDS-related interventions: improving the treatment of sexually transmitted diseases (STDs); voluntary counselling and testing (VCT); MTCTP; and providing HAART for people living with AIDS. It assumes that the interventions will be phased in over time as reflected in Table 4.1.

Table 4.1 *Rates of phase-in for the HIV/AIDS prevention and treatment interventions in the ASSA2000 Interventions Model*

Intervention	2001	2002	2003	2004	2005	2006
STD treatment	0%	20%	40%	60%	80%	90%
VCT	0%	20%	40%	60%	80%	90%
MTCTP	10%	30%	50%	70%	85%	90%
HAART	0%	20%	40%	60%	80%	90%

Source: Johnson and Dorrington (2002: 7)

Improving the treatment of STDs

There is evidence that the presence of an untreated STD increases the risk of HIV infection (see Corbett *et al.* 2002; and Chapter 1).[5] Improving the treatment of STDs can thus act as an AIDS prevention intervention. The ASSA2000 Interventions Model assumes that the treatment of STDs in South Africa is improved in the following ways: private practitioners adopt the syndromic management guidelines for STD treatment; herpes simplex virus-2 cases are treated with acyclovir by both public STD clinics and private practitioners; and all drug shortages at public STD clinics are eliminated. The model assumes that only those suffering from the symptoms of STDs (e.g. genital ulcers, discharge, painful urination, pelvic inflammation) are at a higher risk of transmitting or contracting HIV, and that all STD infections occur in the two high-risk groups. Rates of incidence for STD symptoms were set so that the model reproduced the levels of male STD-prevalence observed in the South African demographic and health survey (Johnson and Dorrington 2002: 10).

In the absence of any STDs (other than HIV), the HIV transmission probability per sexual contact is assumed to be 0.2% for males to females, and 0.1% for females to males. In the presence of STD symptoms other than ulcers, these probabilities are assumed to increase to 2% and 1% respectively, and in the presence of ulcers, both probabilities are assumed to increase to 6% (Johnson and Dorrington 2002: 11). In other words, treating STDs reduces the probability of transmission significantly.[6] As can be seen in Figures 4.3 and 4.4, the model predicts that improving the treatment of STDs will help avert new HIV infections. More specifically, it predicts that between 2001 and 2015, 900,000 fewer people would contract HIV if the treatment of STDs was improved. According to the costing exercise presented in Geffen *et al.* (2003: 8–10),[7] this amounts to R2,400 per HIV infection averted.

Voluntary counselling and testing

There is evidence that voluntary counselling and testing (VCT) programmes can be effective in modifying sexual behaviour in developing countries (Merson *et al.* 2000). For this reason, the ASSA2000 Interventions Model assumes that people who have experienced VCT subsequently modify their sexual behaviour – although this improvement is assumed to wear off over time for those who test HIV-negative.[8] A 20% reduction in the improvement in safe-sex behaviour among those who test HIV-negative is built into the model for each year following VCT (Johnson and Dorrington 2002: 13). Combining the results from randomised control trials in Kenya, Tanzania and Trinidad (VCTESG 2000) and European data (de Vincenzi 1994) the model makes the following assumptions about the effectiveness of VCT (see Table 4.2).

It assumes that the number of individuals receiving VCT in a given year, when the VCT programme is fully implemented, will be 4% of untested HIV-positive people, 3% of untested HIV-negative people who are at risk of HIV-infection, and 1.5% of untested people who are not at risk of HIV-infection. These assumptions (which are inevitably arbitrary) generate the same projected rate of HIV prevalence among individuals who have received VCT as that observed by a Natal-based study (Johnson and Dorrington 2002: 13). According to the model, by 2015 VCT would have resulted in a 16% reduction in unsafe sex between discordant couples (i.e. where one partner is HIV-positive and the other is not), of which 11% is accounted for by the reduction in the proportion of sexual contacts that are unprotected, and 5% by a reduction in the frequency of sex.

Table 4.2 *Assumptions about sexual behaviour change following VCT, by HIV status when VCT is received (ASSA2000 Interventions Model)*

	HIV-negative	HIV-positive (pre-AIDS)	HIV-positive (AIDS)
Reduction in the proportion of sex acts that are unprotected	24%	36%	53%
Reduction in the amount of sex	9%	19%	31%

Source: Johnson and Dorrington (2002: 14)

The model predicts that a VCT intervention could prevent 356,000 new HIV infections between 2001 and 2015. According to an accompanying costing exercise, this amounts to a direct cost of R800 per HIV infection averted (Geffen *et al.* 2003).[9] As is clear from Table 4.3, treating STDs has the greatest impact in terms of saving lives (HIV infections averted), followed by MTCTP. However, in terms of cost-effectiveness, the VCT programme requires fewer resources than the other two interventions per HIV infection averted.

Table 4.3 *Summary statistics on the direct cost-effectiveness of individual HIV prevention interventions*

	HIV infections averted (2001–2015)	Direct Cost per HIV infection averted
Treating STDs	884,000	R2,400
MTCTP*	632,000	R3,100
VCT	356,000	R800

* See Chapter 3, Section 3.4

The estimated effectiveness of a VCT programme is, of course, highly sensitive to the percentage of people assumed to make use of it. As Johnson and Dorrington observe:

[A] key success factor for a VCT programme is its ability to encourage people who are at risk of HIV infection to receive the service. Participation is more likely to occur if those who test positive are offered treatment, and antiretroviral programmes may therefore achieve substantial reductions in high-risk behaviour if coupled with VCT (2002: 15–16).

This raises the important point about the link between providing HAART to those with AIDS, and AIDS prevention interventions.

4.2 The impact of HAART

HAART entails a 'cocktail' of three drugs, typically entailing at least one nucleoside analogue reverse transcriptase inhibitor (NRTI) and one non-nucleoside reverse transcriptase inhibitor (NNRTI).[10] Both sets of drugs interfere with the reverse transcriptase enzyme, which is crucial for the early stage of reproduction of the AIDS virus. NNRTIs attach themselves directly to the enzyme, and NRTIs are incorporated into the DNA strand created by the enzyme, thereby halting further growth of the sequence. The net result is that the reproduction of the AIDS virus is slowed dramatically (viral-loads typically fall to undetectable levels), thus giving the immune system a chance to recover.

The internationally recommended HAART regimen entails two 'lines' of treatment – i.e. two different triple therapy cocktails. This is in order to address problems related to toxicity, resistance and treatment failure. When modelling the impact of treating AIDS with HAART, the ASSA2000 Interventions Model assumes that (two-line) triple therapy is made freely available to adults who are HIV-positive and have experienced AIDS-defining symptoms (or whose CD4 counts are below 200/ul). For children, it is assumed that triple therapy is initiated if the child is experiencing AIDS-defining symptoms, or if their CD4 percentage is below 15% (Johnson and Dorrington 2002: 19). The multi-stage model used to determine overall rates of mortality and morbidity is represented in Figure 4.2. The impact of providing HAART is modelled as providing an extra stage of life for people with AIDS.

The model draws on a wide range of medical literature and information from Somerset Hospital (Cape Town) and the MSF clinic in Khayelitsha (an African township in Cape Town) in order to derive the parameters used to shift people between the various stages, and to estimate the associated mortality and morbidity of people in the different stages. The MSF data is particularly useful as it provides information about the costs and benefits of providing HAART to people living in poor areas. The parameter estimates

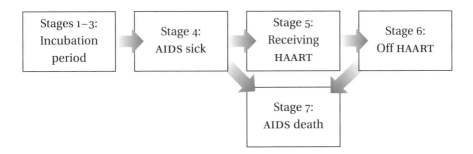

Figure 4.2 *The multi-stage model of disease progression (ASSA2000 Interventions Model)*
Source: Johnson and Dorrington (2002: 19)

are summarised in Table 4.4. Information concerning background sources can be found in Johnson and Dorrington (2002). The model assumes that all those receiving HAART also experience VCT, and hence are subject to

Table 4.4 *Assumptions on mortality, morbidity and infectivity after initiation of HAART (ASSA2000 Interventions Model)*

Parameter	Value
Adult probability of death in the first six months on HAART	8.2%
Per annum thereafter	5.8%
Probability of adult discontinuing HAART in the first six months on HAART	9.1%
Per annum thereafter	5.8%
Child probability of death in the first six months on HAART	9.6%
Per annum thereafter	11.4%
Probability of child discontinuing HAART in the first six months on HAART	13.7%
Per annum thereafter	5.8%
Mortality rate once off treatment	As for untreated AIDS
Reduction in AIDS morbidity on HAART for adults and children	75%
Morbidity rate once off treatment	As for untreated AIDS
Reduction in viral load while on HAART	1.76 logs
Reduction in infectivity per log reduction in viral load	67%
Viral load once off treatment	As for untreated AIDS

Source: Johnson and Dorrington (2002: 20–1).

the same assumptions about sexual behaviour change as discussed in Section 4.1.

The model assumes a phased roll-out of HAART rising to 90% by 2006 (see Table 4.1). Given this and the other assumptions driving the numbers of people on HAART, it is predicted that the number of HAART patients will level off in 2015 at 2.7 million in the non-medical scheme population, and at 260,000 in the medical scheme population.[11] The assumption of a 90% roll-out is almost certainly unrealistic as many people will fail to realise that they have AIDS and seek appropriate treatment and others may be deterred from seeking treatment because of ignorance, social stigma or for more mundane practical reasons. The 90% roll-out figure should thus be regarded as an extreme end of the likely pressure that would be brought to bear on the public sector if a large-scale national HAART programme was implemented.

Figure 4.3 shows the number of HIV infections averted under the different AIDS interventions discussed so far. No overlap is assumed between the programmes, i.e. each intervention is evaluated as if it is the only one in existence. This assumption is relaxed in Section 4.4, which discusses the costs and benefits of expanding the set of prevention interventions to

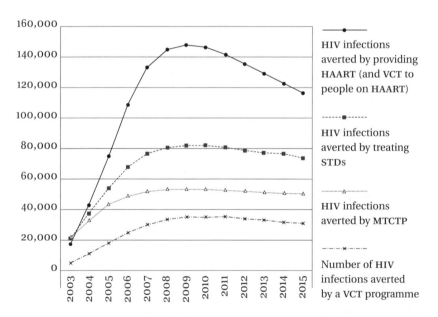

Figure 4.3 *HIV infections averted by the different individual HIV/AIDS prevention and treatment interventions (ASSA2000 Interventions Model)*

include a HAART programme. As can be seen from Figure 4.3, the HAART programme is modelled as being highly effective at preventing new infections. This is because of the reduced infectivity of people on HAART, and because of the assumed impact of the VCT associated with the HAART programme on sexual behaviour change. The impact of HAART on new infections is in large part a product of the assumption that the HAART programme reaches 90% of the HIV-positive people in Stage 4. The model shows that reducing viral loads (and encouraging sexual behaviour change) in a large cohort of HIV-positive people can have a major impact on the course of the pandemic. The impact of HAART on sexual behaviour is explored in more depth in Chapter 5.

Figure 4.5 shows the numbers of AIDS cases (i.e. people who are AIDS-sick) that are projected under the different prevention and treatment scenarios. The VCT and MTCTP interventions reduce the number of AIDS-sick cases over time by reducing the number of HIV-infections. The HAART intervention reduces the number of AIDS-sick cases by treating people with AIDS and by reducing the number of new HIV infections (as described above). In the absence of any prevention or HAART treatment intervention, the number of AIDS cases is likely to peak at 1.24 million in 2010. Implementing a HAART programme (with VCT for those on HAART) reduces the incidence of AIDS-sickness, but because of the increasing numbers of people on HAART, the overall number of AIDS cases increases to a peak in 2015. The figure also shows that about a million deaths would be averted between 2001 and 2015 if a HAART intervention is added to a set of AIDS prevention interventions.

The direct cost of providing HAART

A HAART treatment intervention is the most expensive (in terms of direct costs) of all the HIV/AIDS interventions discussed so far. This is because the cost of antiretroviral medication is so high – even when using the same generic medication purchased by MSF from Brazil. Prices also vary depending on whether patients are on their first-line or second-line treatment.[12] Other costs of HAART include the cost of medical personnel and the costs of lactate dehydrogenase, CD4, full blood count, and differential and amylase tests (Geffen *et al.* 2003: 14–5). Most of the information concerning the time spent by medical personnel in a HAART programme is drawn from the experience of MSF in Khayelitsha.

The costing exercise assumes that patients in their first year of treatment are on a first-line regimen (AZT, Lamivudine, Nevirapine). The

ASSA2000 Interventions Model assumes there is a 20.6% chance of a patient moving to second-line treatment (Didanosine, Stavudine, Lopinavir, Ritonavir) each subsequent year. Once patients move to a second line regimen, they are assumed to remain there until the model removes them from the HAART programme (in line with the assumptions listed in Table 4.4). The costing model also includes a wastage factor of 5% and a 20% additional care factor to account for those patients who require additional care (e.g. due to serious side effects, treatment failure, inadequate recovery, psychological factors, special medicine needs etc. (Geffen *et al.* 2003: 15–16).[13]

This standardised (rather than individual) approach to delivering HAART is in line with recommendations for HAART programmes in resource-poor settings (Weidle *et al.* 2002; Harries *et al.* 2001; Farmer *et al.* 2001; WHO 2002) and is consistent with the assumptions used by the South African government's Joint Health and Treasury Task Team when estimating the cost of a HAART programme for South Africa (2003). It allows for the assessment of suspected drug reactions and can be implemented as part of a programme in which many patients can be treated under the direction of fairly few physicians (Weidle *et al.* 2002: 2262).

The total bill for a HAART programme for the entire period 2003–2015 is just over R125.1 billion. This will fund 21.5 million person years of treatment at an average annual cost per person of about R6,000. As a result of the programme, about 1.5 million new HIV infections will be averted, which amounts to a programme cost of about R83,000 per HIV infection averted. Thus even though the HAART programme averts many more HIV infections than the prevention interventions (see Figure 4.3), the cost of the drugs and related medical expenditure is so high that the cost per infection averted is two orders of magnitude greater than that for VCT on its own. Although a HAART programme has strong preventive elements, ultimately its benefits should also be measured in terms of outputs such as longer life expectancy, fewer orphans etc.

One way of grappling with the issue of the costs and benefits of a HAART programme is to look at the impact of adding a HAART treatment intervention to a set of AIDS prevention interventions. So far, the analysis has looked at each intervention in isolation. This has the effect of inflating the total bill for HAART because if a HAART programme was introduced in addition to HIV prevention programmes, then there would be 207,000 fewer people on HAART in 2015 than there would be if a HAART treatment-only programme was implemented. It thus makes sense to look at the costs of adding a HAART treatment programme to a set of prevention programmes. Section 4.3 looks at the impact of three different scenarios: no intervention; a prevention intervention (including VCT, improved treatment of STDs, and implementing MTCTP); and a prevention plus HAART intervention.

4.3 The cost of AIDS interventions

Figure 4.4 shows the ASSA2000 Interventions Model's estimated impact of the various scenarios on the cumulative number of HIV infections averted and AIDS deaths averted. The figure shows clearly that prevention programmes can significantly reduce the level of HIV infection in society, but that a national HAART programme has the greatest impact in terms of averting AIDS deaths, while also manifesting a strong preventive element. An AIDS intervention programme that combines prevention *and* HAART treatment has the best outcomes in terms of saving and prolonging life. Figure 4.5 shows the impact of three scenarios (no intervention, prevention only, and prevention plus HAART) on AIDS cases and AIDS mortality. The projected numbers for the year 2015 are indicated on the graph.

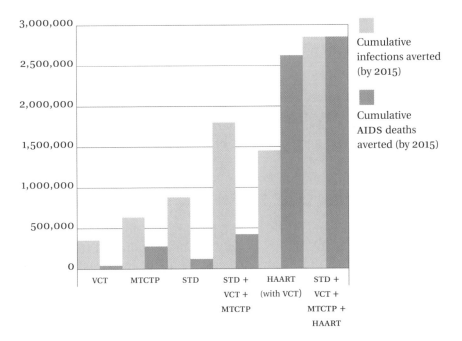

Figure 4.4 *Cumulative HIV infections averted by the different intervention scenarios between 2002 and 2015*

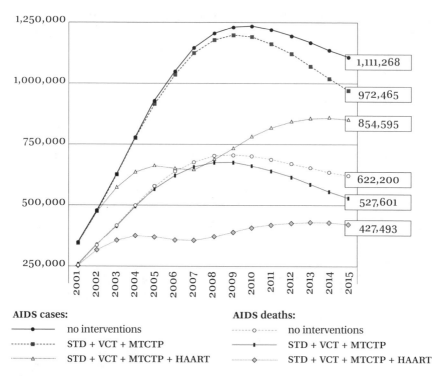

AIDS cases:

—•— no interventions

------■------ STD + VCT + MTCTP

.........△......... STD + VCT + MTCTP + HAART

AIDS deaths:

------○------ no interventions

—|— STD + VCT + MTCTP

.........◇......... STD + VCT + MTCTP + HAART

Figure 4.5 *AIDS cases and AIDS deaths under various scenarios (ASSA2000 Interventions Model)*

What are the costs of these different interventions? Table 4.5 summarises the total cost between 2002 and 2015 of two different scenarios (VCT+ MTCTP+STD, and VCT+MTCTP+STD+HAART) in 2001 prices. A detailed description of the information and assumptions used in estimating the cost of the different scenarios can be found in Geffen *et al.* (2003). Total cost includes an estimate for additional infrastructure (e.g. counselling rooms and site management costs)[14] and public education that would be required for a successful roll-out of an AIDS prevention and treatment intervention. Although these estimated costs could be increased (e.g. by assuming that a higher proportion of HAART patient visits are with doctors), they are reasonable given the evidence that HAART has been successfully piloted in resource-poor settings elsewhere in the world (MSF 2003; Farmer *et al.* 2001; Ramotlhwa 2003; Boulle 2003).

Note that total costs for VCT and MTCTP are lower in the scenario that includes HAART, than for the scenario that does not. This is because of the impact of HAART on reducing the number of new HIV infections (and hence on the need for VCT and MTCTP). The total cost of an STD programme, however, rises as a result of including HAART. This is because the number of sexually active people will rise (as HAART patients live longer and remain sexually active), thus increasing the demand for STD treatment.

Table 4.5 includes an upper- and lower-bound cost estimate for AIDS-related hospitalisation costs. The upper-bound estimate was based on information from Baragwanath Hospital of the costs of treating people at different stages of AIDS-illness (Kinghorn *et al.* 1996; Karstaedt *et al.* 1996). The assumptions are displayed in Table 4.6. The estimate assumes that all people who need medical attention for AIDS-related illnesses will in fact receive it – i.e. it is assumed that no rationing takes place in the public sector with regard to treating people with AIDS.

These upper-bound hospital costs are almost certainly too high – and are substantially higher than the hospitalisation costs estimated by the Joint Health and Treasury Task Team (2003). The cost estimates used in the modelling work reported here were drawn from a major urban hospital providing a full range of treatment and are thus likely to overestimate the average cost in South Africa of treating opportunistic infections (because access to quality health care varies throughout the country: see Table 2.5).[15] It is, unfortunately, very difficult to obtain good estimates of the average cost of treating opportunistic infections in public hospitals. Nevertheless, there are reasons to believe that this estimate may be unrealistic when generalised to the whole of South Africa. According to World Bank data, the cost per patient per year of treating opportunistic infections ranges from $359 in low-income developing countries to $698 in higher-income developing countries (cited in Haacker 2001: 9). This higher-income developing country estimate is roughly a third of the treatment costs estimated here – thus suggesting that the average (upper-bound) treatment costs for opportunistic infections (as indicated in Table 4.6) may be too high. The total upper-bound cost estimate in Table 4.5 (based on Table 4.6) implicitly assumes that all people needing treatment for AIDS-related opportunistic infections are able to obtain the same level of treatment as that achieved in Baragwanath in the mid-1990s. The World Bank figure (which is about two thirds lower) assumes, implicitly, a much lower average level of care provided in public hospitals for the treatment of AIDS-related opportunistic infections.

In recognition of this probable overestimate, Table 4.5 also includes a 'lower-bound' estimate of hospitalisation costs which is approximately one third the value of the upper-bound estimate. The actual costs (which are impossible to ascertain with any level of precision) probably lie somewhere within this large range. This is unsatisfactory, but unavoidable.

Table 4.5 *Average annual cost of AIDS intervention scenarios (with and without HAART) plus hospitalisation costs between 2002 and 2015 (R million)*

	VCT+STD+MTCTP	VCT+STD+MTCTP +HAART
MTCTP	R135	R113
VCT	R20	R17
Improved treatment of STDs	R103	R112
HAART	R0	R9,883
Additional infrastructure, public education and condom distribution	R331	R347
Total direct costs	R589	R10,472
Public hospitalisation costs (upper and lower bound)*	R33,840–R11,167	R28,196–R9,305
Total costs (direct cost plus upper- and lower-bound hospitalisation costs)	R34,429–R11,757	R38,668–R19,777

Source: Costing exercise done in conjunction with the ASSA2000 Interventions Model. See also Geffen *et al.* (2003). * Lower-bound hospitalisation costs reduce the upper-bound costs by two thirds (in line with World Bank data provided in Haacker (2001: 9)). NB: Figures do not add up because of rounding. Total costs are in 2001 prices.

In this regard, it is worth repeating the story (attributed to Lewis Carroll) about the young boy who estimates that there are 1,004 pigs in a field: 'You can't be sure about the four', he is told. 'And you're as wrong as ever,' says the boy, 'it's just the four I can be sure about 'cause they're here, grubbing under the window. It's the thousand I isn't pruffickly sure about' (cited in Boyle 2001: 51). However, if the objective is to estimate with a reasonable degree of certainty that the number of pigs in the field lies between, say, 800 and 1,200, then the need for pinpoint accuracy is reduced. The best we can do with regard to estimating hospitalisation costs is this kind of ballpark (pig-field?) estimate. Leaving them out altogether is even less satisfactory as it effectively ignores a crucial component of the overall cost-benefit calculation. For example, it has been estimated that the Brazilian

HAART programme saved the health sector almost $1.1 billion between 1997 and 2001 by reducing opportunistic infections (Galvao 2002: 1862). As the total cost of the antiretroviral medication amounted to $1.4 billion over the same period (ibid.), it is clear that the savings to the health sector are too important to be ignored. They reduce the net cost of a public-sector programme substantially.

Table 4.6 *Upper-bound hospitalisation costs for patients with HIV*

Stage	Cost per patient per year
Adult Stage 1 and Stage 2	R1,400
Adult Stage 3	R6,600
Adult with AIDS	R18,000
Adult on HAART who has become healthy again	R1,400
Child pre-AIDS	R1,400
Child with AIDS	R18,000

Source: Geffen *et al.* 2003: 24

The total cost in Table 4.5 includes the estimated direct costs of the various programmes *and* the hospitalisation costs experienced by the public sector as a result of the AIDS pandemic (assuming no rationing takes place). As argued above (and in Chapter 3), the hospital costs of HIV-positive people must be included in any estimate of the *net* costs of an HIV/AIDS prevention plus HAART scenario. With regard to the cost of MTCTP, it was argued that once total health costs (i.e. the costs of MTCTP plus the costs of treating HIV-positive children for opportunistic infections) are compared to a no-intervention scenario (i.e. just the cost of treating HIV-positive children for opportunistic infections), then it becomes clear that the government is wasting resources by not introducing MTCTP. This is simply because the costs of treating HIV-positive children are high in relation to the cost of preventing them from becoming HIV-positive in the first place.

Does the same story hold for an AIDS treatment intervention? The Brazilian figures cited above suggest that savings on hospitalisation are substantial ($1.1 billion) but not sufficient to outweigh the costs of the drugs ($1.4 billion).[16] The South African case is likely to be similar. As can be seen from Table 4.5, total hospitalisation costs are lower in the intervention scenario that includes HAART than they are for the one that does not. This is partly because of lower morbidity for people on HAART,[17] but

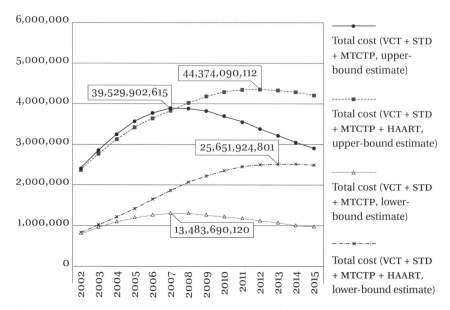

Figure 4.6 *Total costs to the health sector under various intervention scenarios*

mainly because of fewer new HIV infections (and associated hospitalisa-tion costs). Note that the 'saving' is not sufficient to compensate fully for the cost of HAART – hence the total cost of the scenario including HAART is higher than the scenario that does not. In other words, a HAART inter-vention will not 'pay for itself', although it goes a long way towards doing so. The difference in total average annual costs experienced by the health sector between the two scenarios is R4.2–R8 billion (for the upper- and lower-bound estimates). This net increase needed to expand an AIDS intervention to include HAART treatment is less than the R10 billion a year needed to resource a HAART intervention. This is because the HAART intervention is able to claw back a substantial proportion of the resources spent on it through lower hospitalisation expenditure, and lower spending on VCT and MTCTP.

Figure 4.6 shows the trajectory of total health sector costs (i.e. the cost of the interventions plus the cost of treating opportunistic infections) over time. The top two lines depict the costs of the two scenarios assuming the upper-bound hospitalisation costs. The figure shows that the total cost for the scenario including HAART is lower than the costs of the scenario without HAART between 2002 and 2007. This is partly because the HAART programme is phased in (starting from 20% in 2002 and rolling out to 90%

in 2006), which means that the drug costs are likewise phased in. It is also partly the result of the fact that the treatment of opportunistic infections for those on HAART is pushed later in time. As shown in Figure 4.5, the number of AIDS cases flattens off and then rises. Costs relating to treating those with full-blown AIDS kick in later, which is why the cost of the scenario with HAART eventually exceeds that of the scenario without HAART.

If we assume a lower-bound estimate for hospital costs, then Figure 4.6 shows that the total cost of the scenario with HAART exceeds that for the scenario without HAART from 2003 onwards. This is because we are assuming a lower level of care for those with opportunistic infections – thus the advantages of averting and deferring these costs are smaller.

Table 4.7 *The difference between an AIDS intervention with and without HAART*

	VCT+STD+ MTCTP	VCT+STD+ MTCTP+HAART	Difference between the two scenarios
Cumulative HIV infections averted (2002–2015)	1,814,000	2,863,000	1,049,000
Cumulative reductions in AIDS deaths (2002–2015)	415,000	2,859,000	2,444,000
Number of maternal orphans in 2015 under age 18	3,108,000	2,195,000	−913,000
Direct cost per HIV infection averted	R5,000	R51,000	R46,000
Total cost (2002–2015)	R165–R482 billion (R323.5 billion)*	R277–R541 billion (R409 billion)*	R112–R59 billion
Total cost per HIV infection averted	R178,300*	R142,900*	R35,400

* *Mid-point of the upper-bound and lower-bound cost estimates in parentheses*

Table 4.7 presents average annual estimates for key variables. If we take the upper-bound estimate for hospital costs, then more HIV infections will be averted, and at a lower average cost, if an AIDS intervention was expanded to include HAART. However, if we take the lower-bound hospitalisation cost, then the average cost per HIV infection rises slightly when a HAART programme is added. This is because the 'savings' to the state in terms of fewer opportunistic infection cases is smaller. This means that where a relatively high level of care is provided for HIV-positive people suffering from AIDS-related opportunistic infections, then the cost per life saved will decline if the government introduces a HAART programme.

Note that the argument has only considered the benefits of HAART from the narrow financial perspective of the public health sector. It does not try to put an economic value on the fact that fewer orphans would be created,[18] or on the extra years of life gained by people on HAART, or on the economic value of lives saved through lower rates of HIV transmission. If these benefits had been valued, then the economic case in favour of including HAART as part of a broader HIV intervention would be even stronger. The value of this particular (albeit limited) economic calculus is that it speaks directly to the government budget. The strength of the finding is that *even* within this narrow frame of reference, there is a strong economic case to be made in favour of including a HAART programme.

Confronting the conventional economic wisdom

The above argument appears to fly in the face of conventional wisdom in health economics, which holds that HAART is not cost-effective in developing countries. After summarising various cost-effectiveness studies in sub-Saharan Africa, Marseille *et al.* concluded that 'prevention is at least 28 times more cost-effective than HAART', and that 'the next major increments of HIV funding in sub-Saharan Africa should be devoted mainly to prevention and to some non-HAART treatment and care' (2002: 1851). A more systematic review of existing studies of the cost-effectiveness of HIV/AIDS interventions in Africa (Creese *et al.* 2002) came to similar, but more qualified, conclusions. As the policy implications of this are serious indeed, it is worth considering the differences pertaining to methodology and assumptions between the work presented in this chapter, and that summarised by Marseille *et al.* (2002) and Creese *et al.* (2002).

One of the key differences between the South African study presented here, and most other cost-effectiveness data in Africa, is that total hospital costs associated with AIDS are included in the calculation. The intervention scenario without HAART saves fewer new HIV infections over fourteen years than the scenario that includes HAART (1.8 million as opposed to 2.9 million). But the direct cost differential per HIV infection averted is substantial (R5,000 as opposed to R51,000). If, however, we include the hospital costs associated with AIDS-related illness, then the picture changes significantly – especially where a relatively high level of care is provided for those suffering from AIDS-related opportunistic infections.

It is this additional cost calculation which, as was the case with MTCTP, makes a great deal of difference to the conclusion. The problem with the available African cost-effectiveness studies is that they rarely take these 'cost savings' into account (Creese *et al.* 2002: 1637). Instead, the analysis is presented in terms of direct cost per HIV infection averted and/or direct cost per DALY[19] saved. This is a serious limitation. Strong policy conclusions of the kind made by Marseille *et al.* (2002) about the best way of allocating scarce public resources require that the *full* range of AIDS-related demands on the public health system be considered.

The approach adopted by Marseille *et al.* (2002) effectively looks at cost-effectiveness through the eyes of a donor-driven intervention. The public-sector health costs of treating AIDS-related opportunistic infections simply do not enter into the calculation. While this may be a reasonable assumption to make for those African countries with a limited health infrastructure and limited fiscal resources for fighting the AIDS pandemic, it is not an appropriate starting point for analysing a middle-income economy like South Africa that is already spending money on AIDS-related opportunistic infections. Significant health care resources will continue to be expended on addressing the health needs of people living with AIDS. This must be taken into account in any cost-benefit analysis of an AIDS intervention that includes HAART. The modelling exercise reported here indicates that when the costs of treating AIDS-related opportunistic infections are included, the case for including HAART is compelling.

A second problem with Marseille *et al.*'s (2002) approach is the inadequate manner in which it deals with the link between prevention and (HAART) treatment. In their estimate of the cost of treatment, they assume that HAART patients receive no monitoring, testing and counselling (2002: 1852). They assume this as part of a misguided attempt on their part to lower the total costs of a HAART intervention (thus, in their view, biasing the case in favour of HAART). However, in a full modelling exercise, such as that conducted in the ASSA2000 Interventions Model, the fact that those obtaining treatment are also required to undergo VCT has a major impact on sexual behaviour change. The ASSA2000 Interventions Model shows that if you add to the overall cost of a HAART programme the requirement that HAART patients undergo VCT, then the savings (in terms of averting new HIV infections) will pay for the VCT many times over. In other words,

Marseille *et al.* bias their cost calculation heavily *against* HAART by not requiring VCT, and by failing to trace the full demographic benefits of this additional exposure to VCT.

As discussed above, it is precisely the access to VCT (which we assume is necessarily part of a HAART programme) that delivers benefits in terms of additional HIV infections averted. Marseille *et al.* are dismissive of this possibility, saying that there is no quantitative data supporting it (2002: 1853). They accept that there may be a prevention dividend, but are sceptical about its strength. They are also sceptical about the net preventive benefits of lower viral loads.[20] In short, they do not believe that the preventive benefits of HAART are worth taking seriously. Creese *et al.*, in their review of the cost-effectiveness literature, appear to support this position by suggesting that there are no 'public good' and unknown 'externality' benefits for society of providing HIV-positive individuals with HAART (2002: 1641). Such a conclusion can only be based on the assumption that there are no net prevention benefits of a HAART programme.

There are two reasons why the benefits of prevention activities are likely to be substantially enhanced in the presence of a (HAART) treatment programme. Firstly, more HIV-positive people will get counselled and their viral loads will be lowered as a result of HAART. This will result in a fall in HIV transmission. Secondly, more people are likely to come forward and be tested and counselled if there is hope of treatment. As De Cock *et al.* note, 'the advent of therapy in industrialised countries has greatly increased motivation for people to be tested for HIV, and has reduced stigma associated with the disease' (2002: 68). Farmer *et al.* likewise found that the provision of HAART in rural Haiti resulted in a greater demand for testing and opportunity for counselling (2001: 405).

There are those, however, who worry that the presence of a HAART treatment programme will result in people becoming less fearful of HIV-infection and therefore starting to practise riskier sex (see e.g. Marseille *et al.* 2002). The source of this concern is the hypothesis that in higher-income countries, HAART may have contributed to the increase in risky sexual behaviour among a minority of men who have sex with men (MSM). How we grapple with the relationship between prevention and treatment is of great methodological importance. Should we hypothesise that any increase in risky behaviour among MSM is because of HAART – and then, on the basis of this hypothesis, conclude that African heterosexuals will probably respond in the same way? Or should we look at the existing studies of the relationship between VCT and behaviour change in Africa, and work on the basis of that? Furthermore, should we assume that the benefits of lower viral loads among HAART patients will be overwhelmed by behavioural problems and longer life expectancy, or should we model this explicitly and see what the outcome is?

The issue of behaviour change, VCT and HAART is dealt with in more detail in Chapter 5. At this point, suffice it to say that there is no empirical basis to assume that a presumed sexual subcultural response among some members of the gay community in advanced capitalist countries is likely to be replicated in a heterosexual pandemic in Africa. While it is true that the preventive benefits of VCT do not impact on all people in the same way, and do not remain constant over time, the challenge is to model these impacts – not to ignore the issue because of its complexity.

The ASSA2000 Interventions Model is well placed to consider the link between AIDS prevention and treatment. As can be seen in Tables 4.2 and 4.4, the model includes a range of parameters (drawn from existing empirical studies) capturing the impact of VCT on behaviour change, and the impact of lower viral load and longer life expectancy of people on HAART. In other words, the model already captures the uneven impact of VCT on behaviour (and assumes that the beneficial impact of VCT wears off over time for HIV-negative people).[21] It also captures the fact that lower viral loads are counter-balanced to some extent by longer life expectancy.

What are the budgetary implications?

Most cost-effectiveness calculations of AIDS interventions are designed to help answer the question: how should the marginal dollar (or Rand) be allocated in order to save the greatest number of lives. This central economic question is a very useful one to ask when resources are absolutely constrained. However, as argued in Chapter 1, this seemingly technical question is shot through with both implicit and explicit moral judgements. If the only objective was to design an AIDS-intervention strategy which saved the most lives for the least amount of money, then one response might be to deny HIV-positive people access to the public health system altogether! This could be done on the grounds that the few extra DALYs saved by treating their opportunistic infections are not worth the extra cost. The huge bill for hospitalisation costs (see Tables 4.5 and 4.6) would then be reduced significantly. Once this decision was made, the next step would be to consider which intervention saves the most lives for the least amount of money. As indicated in Table 4.3, this would be a VCT intervention. Once this programme had been fully rolled out, any additional resources would then be allocated to treating STDs, and then only if there was still cash available into MTCTP and then, finally, into HAART.

One of the problems with this line of logic is that it leads to a brutalising vision of society without ever questioning the very framework that made the logic necessary in the first place – i.e. the budget constraint. The analysis starts with a constraint: you have limited resources, how should you manage the trade-offs? This is a reasonable starting point if you are in a Crimean War field hospital with no option other than to practise triage. But it is an inappropriate metaphor if used to deflect attention from the larger, prior, question: 'how much would it cost South Africa to implement a full-scale prevention and treatment programme?' As argued in Chapter 1, there is a role for economic analysis to pose these larger questions in order to facilitate social dialogue over the costs and benefits of responding to the AIDS pandemic in ways which promote justice and social solidarity.

Posing this big question, however, immediately raises a further question: what are the implications for the budget? According to the estimates reported in Table 4.7, a full AIDS prevention and treatment intervention would cost between R277 billion (lower-bound estimate) and R541.4 billion (upper-bound estimate) over the period 2002 to 2015. This amounts to an average of R19.8 billion or R38.7 billion respectively per year over the period. Given that South Africa's consolidated national and provincial expenditure on health was R28 billion in 2001/2, this still amounts to a large required increase in government expenditure on health – especially when we consider the upper-bound estimate. Is it affordable?

Firstly, it is important to note that some of the hospitalisation costs included in the total cost estimates are already being borne by the public health sector. According to a department of health report, 12.5% of the total health budget is currently being spent on the costs of hospitalising AIDS patients (2001: 3). If so, then according to the demographic and costing model presented in this chapter, only 20–50%[22] of HIV-positive people are obtaining the treatment they need. If we were to expand government health spending to include the full prevention plus HAART programme outlined above (including, of course, non-rationed care for those suffering from opportunistic infections), then the South African treasury would need to raise between R14.1 billion and R31 billion – depending on what assumptions are made about hospitalisation costs.

The gross domestic product (GDP) in 2001 (in current prices) was R983 billion. So we are talking about spending an extra 1.4–3.2% of GDP. South

Africa raised R61 billion in 2001/2 from value-added tax (VAT), which implies that the South African Revenue Services raises about R4.4 billion for each per cent levied by VAT. This means that we would need to raise VAT by between 3 to 7 percentage points in order to fund a full-scale prevention and treatment intervention. Total taxation as a percentage of GDP would thus rise from 24.6% of GDP to a maximum of 27.8%. While this is a large increase (and the macroeconomic implications of it need to be considered seriously before any decision is made to increase taxation), it is worth noting that in comparative terms a tax take of 27.8% of GDP is not out of line with world averages. According to World Bank data, 40 out of the 106 countries for which there is adequate data have tax revenues as a percentage of GDP higher than this.

An increase in VAT is not necessarily the best way to fund this expenditure because poor people consume more of their income than rich people, and thus they pay a higher proportion of their income back to the Receiver of Revenue than rich people through VAT (even taking into account that some basic goods are VAT-exempt). Other means of raising the additional revenue include an increase in income tax, or some combination of different taxes, borrowing, expenditure cuts in other areas (e.g. defence[23]), and applications for grants and other forms of foreign aid and assistance. The illustrative increase in VAT is simply posed here in order to give an easy-to-grasp indication of the broad implications for taxation.

What about rationing?

An alternative approach to the one presented here is to propose a much more modest HAART intervention that treats fewer people. The 2003 Joint Health and Treasury Task Team projection of the cost of a HAART programme for South Africa comprised three alternative scenarios assuming 100%, 50% and 20% coverage respectively. This suggests that the government may have been considering the possibility of rolling out a treatment programme to a fraction of those who need it.

Estimated direct costs in the first year of the 100% coverage scenario are within the amount allocated by the national treasury in the 2003/4 budget for AIDS treatment. This perhaps suggests that the national treasury was 'already planning and preparing for a national programme to provide anti-retrovirals to South Africans' (Hickey and Ndlovu 2003: 2). Two qualifications are, however, necessary. Firstly, given the state president's and the health minister's stance on antiretrovirals, there may be continued political obstacles to implementation. Secondly, given the constraints imposed by the medium-term expenditure framework, it is unlikely that the treasury is contemplating the same kind of national AIDS prevention plus HAART programme discussed in this chapter. Rationing of HAART is thus likely in the short and medium term.

The best publicly available estimate of a rationed approach to HAART is that by Boulle *et al.* (2002). They estimated the cost of providing (single-line only) HAART treatment to 10% of those who become AIDS-symptomatic. They conclude that the total programme costs of treating 107,000 people (in 2007) would be about R409 million. This amounts to about R3,800 per person on HAART. This is just over half of the cost per person on HAART in 2007 (i.e. R6,200) as estimated by the ASSA2000 Interventions Model because Boulle *et al.* assume only one line of treatment.

In many respects, the data used by Boulle *et al.* are consistent with the data presented here. They do not, however, include a link between treatment and prevention, and they assume a much more limited treatment regimen. The major strategic difference between their approach and the one presented here is, however, the scale of the intervention. Rather than start with an estimate of what is required in terms of treatment, they start with what they think is 'feasible' or 'affordable' given 'existing budget constraints'. It was, in other words, an attempt to get a treatment foot-in-the-door by asking for less resources – rather than spelling out what society needs to consider spending in order to provide HAART to all who need it. Instead of challenging society to fund a full-scale programme, their approach explicitly assumes that this line of action is likely to be counterproductive. They start with the existing level of health spending, treat it as an absolute constraint, and then ask for a marginal shift of resources in favour of treating a limited number of people.

They are not alone in advocating this kind of approach. For example, Haacker (2001) estimates that total HIV-related health services plus HAART for 30% of those who need it would cost about 1.4% of the GDP in South Africa. This, according to Haacker, is affordable. However, as Geffen has pointed out, 'it seems reasonable to ask why aiming for 100% coverage of the HIV-positive population ... at less than 5% of GDP should be fiscally unsound' (2002: 3).

The important word here is 'reasonable'. As argued in Chapter 1, 'reasonableness' is central to decision making among citizens about how best to formulate and achieve social priorities. There is no magic formula as to what is, or is not, 'affordable'. There are always budget constraints and trade-offs – but the size and allocation of the government budget is far more flexible than implied by certain brands of technical economic discourse. Seekings (2003a) cites examples of the discourse of unaffordability used during every successive debate over the expansion of South Africa's welfare system since the 1920s. Once the welfare policy had become entrenched, what had previously been regarded as 'unaffordable' became an accepted part of government responsibility to its citizens. This was the case with the introduction of non-contributory old-age pensions for white and coloured people in 1928, and its extension to Indians and Africans in 1944. South African society needs to grasp the nettle concerning what is required to address the AIDS pandemic, and how to pay for it. This is a decision that requires social reflection and debate. It should not be made by stealth through some limited and narrow intervention which does not spell out the costs in terms of how many lives are not saved as a result of opting for the cheaper, less radical, intervention.

The other, obvious, problem with a rationing strategy is how will the rationing take place? According to what criteria should HAART be allocated to people who need it? For example, the Western Cape government generated a debate within AIDS-advocacy circles when it was announced in June 2003 that the province had sufficient resources to provide HAART to children.[24] But why treat children first? According to DALY-type calculations (which give greater weight to years of life lived by adults than by children) one should treat adults first – particularly those who are breadwinners with large numbers of dependents. But if breadwinners are to be prioritised, then this effectively transforms the income gap between the employed and the unemployed into a hard division between access to life-prolonging medication and early death (see also Chapters 6 and 7).

South Africa is a signatory to the 1990 UN Convention on the Rights of the Child. One of the principles is to 'put children first'. However, this does not necessarily mean treating children ahead of adults. After all, 70% of children born to HIV-positive mothers will be born HIV-negative. Treating mothers thus prevents these children growing up as orphans (and lowers infant mortality rates), and treating mothers and fathers helps protect the income-earning capacity of households. Such benefits to children of treating adults need to be weighed up against the benefits to individual HIV-positive children of receiving HAART.

In short, it is not clear what principle is being adopted by a 'treat children first' rationing strategy. There may be practical advantages to this policy in that the infrastructure is available (all pregnant women in the Western Cape have access to VCT and children are reachable through the immunisation programme). However, it is far from clear whether these practical advantages outweigh the practical advantages of treating entire families – and rolling out the treatment to more sites as more resources become available. There are also ethical problems involved in providing life-prolonging treatments to children while denying it to mothers and fathers. It sends out a message that only the 'innocents' deserve treatment – thus contributing further to the stigmatisation of AIDS. Treating all lives as equal is a preferable strategy, especially from a human rights perspective.

It is likely that rather than announce an explicit rationing strategy, the government may simply choose to 'roll-out' a HAART treatment programme to very limited numbers of sites and/or at a far slower rate than desired by AIDS activists. While it is inevitable that a national HAART programme will have to start in urban hospitals (because this is where the best capacity exists to deliver such a programme), there is no necessary reason why capacity cannot steadily be generated elsewhere – thus facilitating a broader roll-out (see discussion in Section 4.4 below). Unless this happens, an AIDS treatment programme will favour those living close to hospitals and will exacerbate urban-rural differentials.

Another way of rationing HAART is to allow doctors to prescribe it, but not to embark on a large-scale publicity campaign. If large numbers of HIV-positive people fail to get tested, and simply die of opportunistic infections, then the actual demand for HAART will be far lower than that projected here. This chapter presents the 'worst-case' scenario for the government in terms of HAART programme costs. Actual demand is likely to be far lower because of failure to test, reluctance to accept HAART, fear of stigma, etc. If the government embarks on a treatment programme as a low-priority and low-visibility policy, then take-up rates are likely to remain low, thus effectively rationing HAART. Under this scenario TAC and other advocacy groups are likely to remain active even in the presence of a government-funded treatment programme.

4.4 'Scaling-up' the use of HAART in the public sector

During 2003, as it became more and more likely that the government would be forced to introduce HAART in the public sector, the AIDS policy debate shifted towards the challenges involved in 'scaling-up' a treatment programme. This included the need for Brazilian-style negotiations with the large pharmaceutical companies over the prices of antiretrovirals, and a concerted effort to support the domestic production of generics, under either voluntary or compulsory licences.[25] The launch in August 2003 of South Africa's first generic antiretroviral drug (containing stavudine) under a voluntary licensing agreement with Bristol-Myers Squibb was a particularly welcome development.[26] As econometric analysis of anti-retroviral price trends reveals, reliance on 'corporate philanthropy' does not guarantee long-term sustainability of lower-differential pricing, and that the introduction of generic competition remains an essential factor for price decreases (Lucchini *et al.* 2003). Ensuring that testing facilities (to conduct CD4 cell count tests, viral loads, etc.) expand in line with demand from the health sector is a further challenge for the private-sector and/or public-private partnerships.[27]

The implications for the health sector of a full-scale national treatment programme are immense (Schneider 2003). The costing exercise presented here included the cost of additional doctors, nurses and counsellors. Hiring extra staff is necessary in order to ensure that the introduction of a HAART programme does not drain much needed financial and human resources from other parts of the health system. Additional infrastructure (e.g. consultation rooms) was also included in the costing exercise, although it is possible that further unexpected costs may be incurred. For example, the theft of antiretrovirals proved to be an unexpected problem in Botswana, with the result that they had to be stored in the same way as narcotics – thus posing additional expenses on the health system (Ramotlhwa 2003). Presumably once HAART programmes become available elsewhere in Southern Africa, theft will become less of a problem.

Most importantly, a national HAART programme needs to be rolled out in a way that improves the functioning of the existing health care system – i.e. as a vehicle for upgrading (rather than undermining) it. This is why it is so important to stress the additional resource requirements associated with a treatment roll-out. In addition, the management and monitoring of HAART patients needs to be integrated with other programmes, most obviously with the treatment of tuberculosis, but also with that of other opportunistic infections. It is also important to address the shortage of skilled personnel in the health system and to provide the necessary laboratory testing facilities and other support infrastructure (Schneider 2003: 24–8).

Systemic challenges such as these are serious, but not insurmountable. As the deputy director general of health in the Western Cape provincial government argued at an August 2003 workshop on scaling up antiretro-virals in the public sector, the complexity of a HAART intervention should 'not be exaggerated' (Abdullah 2003). By mid-2003, the Western Cape had two and a half years of experience with pilot treatment programmes reaching over 1,000 HAART patients.[28] Abdullah (2003) pointed out that medical staff and volunteers were very keen to introduce a HAART programme in the public health sector, and rolling out treatment would constitute a much needed boost to morale.

Boulle (2003) was similarly optimistic about the prospects of rolling out a HAART programme in the Western Cape. He argued that the Khayelitsha pilot project shows how antiretroviral interventions can be used to improve access to health services, and to graduate the level of care (e.g. from MTCTP, to the treatment of opportunistic infections, to providing HAART, and now integrating the management of TB and AIDS. He argued that a more nurse-centred HAART programme is possible.

One of the most encouraging lessons of the Western Cape pilot pro-grammes is that HAART patients are not overwhelmed by the 'complexity' of the treatment intervention and understand the need to adhere to the drug regimen. Good adherence requires adequate counselling and other support programmes, but the pilot projects show that good adherence is possible in resource-poor settings (Abdullah 2003; Coetzee and Boulle 2003). This is consistent with evidence from Cote d'Ivoire, Uganda and Senegal (Moatti et al. 2002). Recent evidence from Gauteng points to similar conclusions (Mlongo 2003). Coetzee and Boulle point out that the clinic waiting room becomes a 'support area', with patients discussing with each other adherence issues and problems relating to overcoming side effects (2003). In addition, HAART patients in Khayelitsha have become powerful community advocates of treatment, which has helped reduce stigma and encourage disclosure in the area (Coetzee and Boulle 2003). The Botswana experience also indicates that HAART helps 'break the cycle of denial and infection', thus strongly supporting prevention (Ramotlhwa 2003).

There is, of course, always the question of whether the success of pilot projects can be replicated on a larger scale as the treatment programme rolls out in 2004 and 2005. In this regard, the experience of Botswana is highly instructive. The national treatment programme was initially concentrated in four strategically located sites (Gaberone, Francistown, Maun and Serowe) and then expanded to include three army facilities and two mining hospitals. A further ten hospitals were then identified as addi-tional sites (Ramotlhwa 2003). After 18 months of experience with rolling out HAART, the results were very encouraging: patient follow-up exceeded 90% and complete viral load suppression was recorded in over 85% of patients (Ramotlhwa 2003).

One of the problems with rolling out a HAART programme by starting with well-resourced urban hospitals is that many of those who need access to treatment will not receive it (at least not for some time). There is, in other words, a trade-off between implementing the programme efficiently, and ensuring immediate equitable access. Unfortunately there is little scope for 'balancing' these concerns, because a poorly implemented HAART programme will be of limited benefit to patients, and runs the danger of increasing drug resistance. There is no real alternative other than to start where the capacity exists for effective intervention, and then to expand that capacity as fast as possible to other areas. The challenge, of course, is to allocate sufficient resources for developing this capacity.

4.5 HAART or a disability grant?

The South African government faces significant fiscal exposure to the AIDS pandemic through the welfare system. A government means-tested disability grant of a maximum of R700 a month is available to all 'severely physically and mentally disabled people' older than 18. This includes people living with AIDS. However, there is no clear policy on AIDS-related disability grants: some provinces give the grant to people in Stage 3 of the illness (others restrict access to Stage 4); and some disability grant dispensing points require the grant to be renewed every six months, whereas others – even in the same province – do not have this requirement (Boulle 2003). The situation is thus chaotic and unsatisfactory. Means-tested caretaker grants are available to the caretakers of disabled children (including those affected by AIDS). None of these costs (and associated costs averted if a full-scale prevention and treatment programme was implemented) have yet been included in the analysis.

In 2001, 643,000 people were receiving disability grants, which, in the opinion of Van der Berg and Bredenkamp, was a surprisingly low figure given the eligibility criteria (2002: 50). However, by October 2002, the number of disability grants had risen sharply to 831,271. Simkins observes that this 'probably reflects an increase in take-up rates as well as the rising number of people disabled by the development of full-blown AIDS' (2003: 8). Between April 2001 and June 2002, the number of child care dependency grants also rose sharply from 24,073 in March 2000 to 30,628 in July 2001 and then to 49,265. This trend may also be in part a result of 'the

emergence of claims for children seriously ill as a result of HIV infection'
(ibid. 11).

Using data from the ASSA2000 model, Simkins estimates that the
number of non-AIDS-disabled and AIDS-disabled (i.e. those with full-
blown AIDS) in 2002 was 825,280 and 270,811 respectively (ibid. 8). In
order to match these figures with the number of grants actually paid,
Simkins assumes that the take-up rate for the disability grant by the non-
AIDS-disabled was 92.5%, and 25% for the AIDS-disabled.[29] Assuming a
constant take-up rate for the non-AIDS-disabled, and a rise in the take-up
rate for the AIDS-disabled from 25% to 75% in 2012, Simkins estimates that
the number of disability grants will rise to 1,236,847 in 2010.[30] The costs to
the government will rise from R6.4 billion to R9.5 billion as a result (ibid.
9). Costs associated with care dependency grants could also increase
substantially as a result of AIDS (Barberton 2000).

If a HAART programme was in place, then those who respond well to
treatment will in many cases (although this seems to vary from province
to province and pay-out point to pay-out point) no longer be eligible for a
disability grant. The government would thus 'save' a significant portion of
this projected increase. The problem with this scenario, however, is that
the loss of the disability grant may have serious financial and other
implications for people living with AIDS. Welfare transfers, like pensions
and disability grants, are important components of household income –
particularly for households at the bottom end of the income distribution
(Seekings 2000).

It is thus to be expected that for many people living with AIDS, the disability grant was a source of great relief. One of the respondents interviewed
as part of a broader study of the impact of AIDS, went as far as to say 'I love
this HIV' because of it. She explained her choice of words as follows:

Yes I like this HIV/AIDS because we have grants to support us ... Before I was staying
with my mother and father and sister, they didn't work. Maybe I was taking three to four
days without food. People discriminated against me and no one came in the house. The
only thing that was helping was my grandmother's pension. We were surviving on that
money. Concerning the illness, our lives are changed completely (quoted in Steinberg
et al. 2002b: 29).

The notion that someone might 'love this HIV' seems shocking. But it is
understandable (albeit in a terrible way) when one considers the desperate circumstances that households can find themselves in when they lack

access to an income earner. Household survey evidence since the mid-1990s has consistently shown a strong relationship between unemployment and poverty (Seekings 2000; Leibbrandt *et al.* 2000; Seekings 2003b). Those households with neither access to a pensioner nor an income earner find themselves in deep poverty. Individuals without the human, social and financial capital needed to obtain a job are particularly disadvantaged (Seekings 2003b). Unemployment rates are especially high among the youth – i.e. those constituencies most devastated by AIDS (see Table 4.8). The advent of a disability grant under such circumstances (as was clearly the case for the respondent quoted above) is a major lifeline for the entire family. The threat of its removal as a result of HAART is thus serious indeed.

On one level it is entirely appropriate that a person should lose the disability grant once they start to enjoy better health as a result of HAART. The individual is now able to work and be a fully functional member of the household. However, in a situation where the desire and the ability to work do not translate into obtaining employment, the matter becomes more ethically problematic. This is the case in South Africa today, where unemployment is high and rising and formal employment has declined

Table 4.8 *Unemployment rates by age and the age distribution of the unemployed in South Africa (October Household Survey, 1999)*

	16–25	26–35	36–45	46–55	56–65	Total
Strict definition (i.e. active job seekers)						
Men	38%	21%	13%	10%	7%	19%
Women	48%	31%	20%	12%	5%	27%
Total	42%	26%	16%	11%	7%	23%
Broad definition (i.e. including discouraged job seekers)						
Men	52%	30%	20%	18%	14%	29%
Women	64%	47%	33%	24%	16%	43%
Total	58%	39%	27%	21%	15%	36%
% who have never worked before						
Unemployed (strict)	80%	62%	45%	40%	39%	64%
Unemployed (broad)	84%	67%	53%	48%	45%	68%

Source: Nattrass 2002

steadily for over a decade (Nattrass 2003a). The South African growth path, which since the 1970s has been characterised by rising capital-intensity, appears to have become even less conducive to employment growth since 1990 (Fedderke and Mariotti 2002). As shown in Figure 4.7, formal manufacturing employment increased marginally in the mid-1990s, but nosedived thereafter. Public-sector employment helped boost overall employment until the mid-1990s, but has, since 1996, contracted alongside private-sector non-agricultural employment. Agriculture has also shed significant numbers of jobs (Simbi and Aliber 2000). The rise in unemployment has resulted in a significant increase in poverty, particularly between 1999 and 2002 (Meth and Dias 2003).

South Africa's welfare system, which is premised on full employment (Nattrass and Seekings 1997), assumes that only the young, the elderly and the disabled are in need of support. Working-age adults are expected to earn their own income, and unemployment insurance is available for a limited period only (and only to those who have contributed to the Unemployment Insurance Fund when they were working). The South African welfare system has thus not been able to respond to the challenge

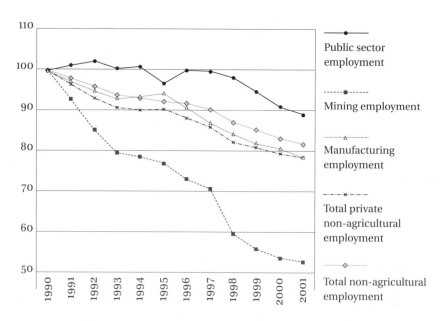

Figure 4.7 *Trends in non-agricultural formal employment in the 1990s (data from the South African Reserve Bank). Index: 1990 = 100.*

of rising long-term unemployment since the mid-1970s. With regard to the unemployed, South Africa's 'welfare net' has a very large hole.

The life chances and living standards of entire households are compromised when working-age adults cannot find employment.[31] According to the government household and labour-force surveys conducted from the mid-1990s onwards, over a third of those who say that they want jobs report that they are out of work.[32] This amounts to about 4.7 million people and it is, without question, a socio-economic crisis of major proportions. If unemployment stagnates or grows, South Africa's already high level of inequality will probably worsen.[33]

Unemployed people who have their health restored by HAART may thus find themselves in a very difficult labour market position. Those who previously had access to a disability grant (but lose it as a result of regaining their health) may find themselves without an income to support themselves. They could thus face a terrible choice: not to take antiretrovirals and keep the disability grant for the short time they have left to live; or take the antiretrovirals, live longer but without an income. Such a choice could result in many people 'yo-yoying' between disability grants and AIDS treatment, with the result that the treatment regimen will be a lot less effective and more conducive to drug resistance (Boulle 2003).

This Scylla versus Charybdis choice is not one that a civilised society ought to be imposing on its citizens. Access to antiretroviral medication should, at the very least, be accompanied by food parcels/welfare relief for those in poverty. It makes no sense to provide someone with life-prolonging medication if they are unable to meet their basic nutritional requirements. One option is to provide people on HAART with a reduced disability grant, rather than remove it altogether. However, this raises the obvious question as to why *all* poor people should not be given a similar grant. As argued in Chapter 7, there are strong grounds for linking a full-scale AIDS prevention and treatment intervention to the introduction of a basic income grant for all South Africans.

5 AIDS, HAART and behaviour change

Chapter 4 reported the results of a demographic modelling exercise which assumed that an AIDS treatment intervention not only extends the lives of those on HAART, but also results in fewer new HIV infections. This is because (as modelled by the ASSA2000 Interventions Model) HIV-positive people are less infectious when they are on HAART, and because more of them will participate in a VCT programme when AIDS treatment interventions are available. The ASSA2000 Interventions Model assumes that people who have experienced VCT subsequently modify their sexual behaviour, although this improvement is assumed to wear off over time for those who test HIV-negative.

The idea that a HAART programme has a strong preventive element is often greeted with scepticism and surprise. The government's Joint Health and Treasury Task Team reflected the conventional wisdom on the topic by stating that there is 'no compelling evidence that antiretrovirals would reduce numbers of new infections' (2003: 18). Any argument to the effect that HAART is likely to prevent new HIV infections thus needs to be developed in more detail.

As noted above, the ASSA2000 Interventions Model relied on several behavioural studies indicating that there is a positive relationship between behaviour change and VCT. But is this a reliable basis for modelling the net behaviour change resulting from HAART? VCT can facilitate shifts towards safer sexual practices, but might not the very availability of HAART itself result in behaviour change in the opposite direction, i.e. by encouraging people to relax their guard and practise less safe sex? Or is it possible that the existence of HAART could promote safer sexual practices by reducing the social marginalisation and stigmatisation of people living with AIDS, thereby making it more likely that HIV-positive people will try not to pass on the disease? As such questions are important, the topic is worthy of specific consideration.

5.1 Does HAART lead to riskier sex?

Those who argue in favour of 'prevention rather than treatment' tend to be sceptical of the prevention benefits of HAART programmes. In particular, they worry about the possibility that HAART treatment may result in an increase in risky sexual behaviour – thus contributing to the spread of AIDS, rather than reducing it. According to Marseille *et al.*:

These dangers are not only theoretical: San Francisco has recently witnessed evidence of increased HIV incidence that may well be linked to misconceptions that HAART is equivalent to a cure and that it eliminates transmission risk by those with HAART-associated viral load reductions. There is some early indication that similar dynamics might operate in less-developed countries. A recently reported 3.7% rise in HIV incidence in Brazil was attributed by the Brazilian ministry of health to decreased condom use in young men who have sex with men. The Health Ministry added that the decline in condom use 'seemed to have started after the introduction' of antiretroviral drug therapy, which Brazil provides for free to all citizens with AIDS. The added survival conferred by HAART may exacerbate these effects (2002: 1854).

The first thing to note about the above quote is the qualified language. The increase in HIV incidence in San Francisco 'may well be linked' to HAART, and the decrease in condom use 'seemed to have started' after HAART was introduced. The argument in large part amounts to conjecture because there is no hard evidence for any causal connection between HAART and increased HIV incidence. The thin evidential base for Marseille *et al.*'s argument is born out by an examination of the sources they cite. Their reference for the Brazilian story is a newspaper report, and for the San Francisco trend it is a short article published in the *Morbidity and Mortality Weekly Report* (Page-Shafer *et al.* 1999). This article reported on the results of a set of surveys conducted by volunteers in the Stop AIDS Project, a San Francisco community-based organisation.

In this study, men who have sex with men (MSM) were approached in clubs, bars, neighbourhoods and outdoor events and asked to respond to peer-administered one page questionnaires. The resulting annual cross-sectional surveys between 1994 and 1997 revealed an increase in anal sex, in unprotected anal intercourse (UAI) and in the number of sexual partners. This was particularly pronounced among younger men. The general increase in recorded risky behaviour was accompanied by a rise in rectal gonorrhea (Page-Shafer *et al.* 1999).

No association is made in this report between HAART and increased risky behaviour (as it was not the subject of the study, and no questions were asked about the link between risk behaviour and motivations for it). Instead, an accompanying 'editorial note' hypothesised about a possible connection between HAART and these reported trends:

The increase in reported risk behaviours and increases in STDs in San Francisco coincide with the expanded availability of effective ART (antiretroviral therapy) in San

Francisco and the United States. Although ART can result in decreased viral load and decreased risk for HIV transmission, advances in HIV treatment and the resulting declines in AIDS deaths in San Francisco and nationally might lead to increased risk behaviour by MSM who perceive that HIV infection can be managed effectively.[1]

Here we have an argument based on the fact that the increase in reported risk behaviour *coincided* with HAART and the supposition that HAART *might* lead to increased risky behaviour. The reference for this theory is a letter published in the *New England Journal of Medicine*. Given that coincidence and hypothesis does not amount to causality, we can conclude that there is no hard evidence cited in the sources used by Marseille *et al.* (2002) to question the preventive benefits of providing HAART. The rise in risky behaviour among surveyed MSM may be the result of selection bias in the set of cross-sectional surveys (discussed in more detail below) or the result of other changes in the environment besides the introduction of HAART – for example, the growth of the Internet. According to a study by McFarlane *et al.* (2000), those who seek sex through the Internet are more likely to be homosexual and to engage in risky sexual behaviour. One could, in other words, just as plausibly suggest that it is the growth of Internet dating among MSM that is the root cause of the rise in risky behaviour among some groups.

Given that coincidence does not amount to causality, studies based on cohorts of HAART patients are better placed to make stronger conclusions about any potential link between AIDS treatment and risky sexual behaviour. However, these kinds of studies are of limited relevance in the sense that they only capture one possible dimension of HAART-related behaviour change, i.e. that experienced by patients on HAART. Nevertheless, they are instructive. A Dutch study of HIV-positive MSM of all ages found that risky sexual behaviour increased in HAART patients once CD4 cell counts had risen and viral loads had dropped to undetectable levels – but that the frequency of unsafe sex was lower again with sustained virological and immunological improvements seen with continued treatment (reported in Stolte *et al.* 2002: 21). This suggests that the increase in risky behaviour among MSM may be temporary. An appropriate policy implication may thus be that care should be taken to counsel people on HAART (particularly young MSM) during the time when they first start to feel the beneficial health impact of HAART – rather than to deny them the chance of obtaining HAART on the assumption that they will respond by increasing their risky behaviour (as implicitly assumed by Marseille *et al.* 2002).

Note also that even if there is an increase in risky sexual behaviour by people on HAART, one cannot draw a straight link between this and increased risk of HIV transmission because of HAART. HAART patients have lower viral loads, and hence are less infectious. As greater risk behaviour and lower infectivity work in opposite directions, the net impact on HIV transmission risk is unclear. However, if the study cited above is anything to go by, the net increased risk of HIV transmission is almost certainly lower for HAART patients – if only because the increase in risky behaviour appears to be temporary and takes place at a time when viral loads are undetectable.

Of greater importance, perhaps, than the behaviour of those on HAART, is the impact of the availability of life-prolonging treatment on attitudes and risk behaviour in the broader population. This is why survey-based studies, such as the San Francisco study cited above, are useful. But these studies, too, have their limitations. An obvious problem with the San Francisco study is that the sample cannot be assumed to be representative of the broader MSM community in the area. This is true also for other international studies that have found increases in sexual risk behaviour among MSM in Holland (Stolte *et al.* 2002), Spain (Perez *et al.* 2002), Canada (CIDPC 2002) and Switzerland (Dubois-Arber *et al.* 2002). These studies recruited their respondents from bars, clubs, gay organisations, gay media and the like. If MSM who have decided to practise safe sex no longer frequent gay clubs (or do so less often), then there will be a strong selection bias in studies that recruit their respondents from such clubs. Studies showing an increase in reported high-risk behaviour could simply be surveying a changing population whose composition reflects an increasing proportion of high-risk individuals.

Likewise, those studies that recruit their respondents from STD clinics (as is the case with the Dutch study cited above) are more likely to be interviewing those who have continued to engage in risky behaviour – rather than those who have changed behaviour and lowered their risk of STD infection. In the absence of other data on the MSM population in Amsterdam, the Dutch study cannot conclude that the increase in STDs and risky behaviour as recorded by STD clinics is representative of MSM in the area.

A recent study in Barcelona compared the results of cross-sectional surveys between 1998 and 2000 of MSM (recruited mainly from saunas, sex shops and pick-up sites in the public parks) in 1998 and 2000. The main finding was that there were no significant changes in HIV prevalence or risky behaviour over the period (Perez *et al.* 2002: 27). However, concern was raised about the minority of respondents who expressed optimism about HAART. Perez *et al.* report that:

Participants who agree that 'HIV-positive persons taking ARV therapy are unlikely to transmit HIV' are 1.9 times more likely to have UAI with casual partners, and those who agree that 'with ARV it is likely to avoid HIV infection after a potential sexual risk exposure' are 1.7 times more likely. Similarly, those who report 'being less afraid of becoming HIV positive' and 'paying less attention to prevention' or 'being less worried if they take sexual risks' are also more likely to have UAI (2002: 27).

Evidence of this kind indicates that there may be a connection between HAART and increased sexual risk behaviour for a minority of MSM. However, commenting on the growing literature of this kind, Laporte notes that 'surveys on knowledge, attitudes and sexual behaviour in the new therapeutic context remain unconvincing' (2002: 15). He argues that the studies published since 1997 show 'an excellent understanding of the benefits and limits of new treatments and a minority of people (less than 10% of all respondents) reporting a decreasing practice of safer sex because of treatment possibilities' (ibid.). He speculates that this minority may comprise those 'who regularly took risks before the introduction of new treatments, thus justifying their behaviours with hindsight' (ibid.). In other words, neither a causal connection (nor its direction) can be established between attitudes to HAART and risky sexual behaviour.

The best available study of the possible relationship between HAART and sexual risk behaviour is that by the International Collaboration on HIV Optimism (2003). MSM were surveyed in 2000 in Australia (Sydney and Melbourne), Canada (Vancouver), England (London) and France (Paris). In all cities, most men were currently employed, around one in five reported having had an STD in the past 12 months, and more than one half said they were in a relationship with another man (2003: 547). The study distinguished between two dimensions of possible 'HIV optimism': one relating to the reduced severity of HIV infection (because HAART boosts the immune system); and the other to reduced susceptibility (because people on HAART are less infectious). To capture both dimensions of HIV optimism, the study asked all MSM to respond to the following statements (2003: 546):
- New HIV treatments will take the worry out of sex.
- If every HIV-positive person took the new treatments, the AIDS pandemic would be over.

- People with an undetectable viral load don't need to worry so much about infecting others with HIV.
- HIV/AIDS is a less serious threat than it used to be because of new treatments.

Table 5.1 *Mean HIV optimism scores between and within cities*

	London (n = 690)		Paris (n = 1,715)		Sydney/ Melbourne (n = 3,120)		Vancouver (n = 357)	
	Mean	95% CI	Mean	95% CI	Mean	95% CI	Mean	95% CI
All men	6.3	6.2–6.4	5.1	5.0–5.2	6.4	6.3–6.5	6.8	6.6–7.0
By HIV status:								
HIV-positive	6.4	6.0–6.8	5.4	5.2–5.6	6.5	6.3–6.7	7.3	6.5–8.1
HIV-negative	6.3	6.1–6.5	5.0	4.9–5.1	6.4	6.3–6.5	6.8	6.6–7.0
Never tested	6.1	5.8–6.4	5.3	5.1–5.5	6.8	6.5–7.1	6.6	5.0–8.2
p (within city)	0.5		<0.001		<0.05		0.5	
By age:								
<30	6.6	6.3–6.9	4.9	4.8–5.0	6.5	6.3–6.7	6.9	6.7–7.1
30–39	6.2	6.0–6.4	5.1	5.0–5.2	6.4	6.3–6.5	6.8	6.6–7.0
>39	6.3	6.0–6.6	5.2	5.1–5.3	6.4	6.3–6.5	–	–
p (within city)	0.05		<0.05		0.7		1	
By sexual risk behaviour:								
UAI with casual partner	6.8	6.4–7.2	5.5	5.3–5.7	7	6.8–7.2	6.7	6.3–7.1
No UAI	6.1	5.9–6.3	4.9	4.8–5.0	6.3	6.2–6.4	6.8	6.5–7.1
p (within city)	<0.001		<0.001		<0.001		0.5	

Source: International Collaboration on HIV Optimism *(2003: 548).* * p values between cities were <0.001 for all variables

Responses were recorded on the following 4-point scale: (1) strongly disagree, (2) disagree, (3) agree, (4) strongly agree. The responses to each question were then added together to get an index ranging from 4 (the respondent strongly disagreed with each statement) to 16 (the respondent strongly agreed with each statement). A score of 8 indicated that on average the respondent disagreed with all four statements (i.e. were not optimistic). As can be seen in Table 5.1, overall mean optimism scores were low (range across cities 5.1–6.8), indicating that most MSM disagreed or disagreed strongly with all four statements. The study notes:

What is striking about this finding is that these gay men were recruited in cities where HAART had been widely available for 4 years at the time of the survey. Despite the dramatic and visible reduction in HIV-related mortality and morbidity in these cities since 1997, only a few gay men expressed 'HIV optimism'. Far from being optimistic, most gay men appeared to be realistic about the benefits of these drugs (International Collaboration on HIV Optimism 2003: 548).

UAI with a casual partner was used as the measure of risky sexual behaviour. The 18–39% of MSM who reported UAI with a regular partner were excluded from the analysis on the grounds that this group is at a lower risk of contracting HIV than those who have UAI with casual partners (International Collaboration on HIV Optimism 2003: 547).

There was no consistent relationship between HIV optimism and HIV status – thus highlighting the heterogeneous nature of gay men's responses to HAART (ibid. 548). In all countries except Canada, mean optimism scores were higher (but still in the pessimistic range) for MSM who reported UAI with a casual partner than for those who did not. However, as the study notes, causality could not be established from this kind of cross-sectional analysis: 'It is impossible to say whether HIV optimism triggered high-risk behaviour or whether treatment optimism was used as a post-hoc rationalisation to justify sexual risk-taking' (International Collaboration on HIV Optimism 2003: 549).

In short, the conventional wisdom that HAART could easily result in a significant increase in risky sexual behaviour among MSM amounts to little more than a 'moral panic'. There is no scientific basis for assuming that the advent of HAART has resulted in increased risk behaviour among MSM in high-income countries. There is even less basis for assuming that a possible behavioural response of a small minority of MSM is likely to be replicated in Africa, where the dynamics of the HIV pandemic are very different. Even if a small minority of MSM have increased the riskiness of their sexual behaviour in response to HAART, we need to know how transportable this is to the African pandemic. The fact that the risk of unprotected intercourse is three times higher for MSM receiving HAART than it is for heterosexuals receiving HAART (Laporte 2002: 15) suggests that the problem in advanced capitalist countries seems to be concentrated among MSM rather than heterosexuals. And, according to a study of

MSM in Amsterdam, recent increases in risky sexual behaviour were lowest among bisexual men and MSM of non-Western nationality (Stolte 2002: 20).

Taken together, this suggests that the problem (to the extent that it exists at all) may be located within a particular sexual subculture – and that this subculture has little obvious relevance for the African pandemic. It is thus an unacceptable leap of logic to argue (as do Marseille *et al.* 2002) that because of a hypothetical link between HAART and risky sexual behaviour (for which there is little, if any, evidence) we should be cautious about introducing HAART in Africa. Indeed, evidence from Côte d'Ivoire indicates that people with access to HAART use condoms more frequently than untreated HIV-positive people (Moatti *et al.* 2002: 100).

5.2 Could *failure* to provide HAART lead to riskier sex?

As observed earlier, the possibility that HAART may lead to increased risk behaviour is often cited by those who are sceptical of the social impact of AIDS treatment. But the alternative – i.e. the impact on behaviour change of *not* introducing HAART – is never considered. The implicit counter-factual for those who oppose HAART is that the failure to provide treatment will have no adverse effects on behaviour. But what if this is incorrect? What if HIV-positive people feel so marginalised and rejected that some of them set out to infect others with the virus?

In this regard, there is reason to believe that a minority of people in South Africa may be spreading HIV deliberately. A survey among Zulu speakers in Durban found that just over 60% of respondents said it was common or very common for people to be spreading AIDS deliberately. Of the respondents, 24% said that they knew people who were spreading HIV deliberately, and a 'small, but important portion' reported that they would spread HIV deliberately if they found they were HIV-positive (Jones and Varga 2001: 31–2). This echoes the results of earlier research among youth in KwaZulu-Natal that young people were adhering to the slogan 'infect one, infect all' (Leclerc-Madlala 1997). As Jones and Varga observe, 'to suggest that a dire need exists for research into the apparent empathetic void, and for identification of a means of addressing it, would be an understatement' (2001: 32–3).

It is impossible to say how many people may be experiencing this 'empathetic void' and opting to spread AIDS deliberately – or why they are behaving in this manner. Leclerc-Madlala (1997) argues that this behaviour stems primarily from a lack of hope and a desire not to die alone. One of her respondents argued as follows:

You lose hope. You know that you'll be rejected; you know you're going to die. All you can do is go off and spread it. It's your only hope knowing that you won't die alone. It's the one thing you have to lean on really (ibid. 369).

Another had more aggressive reasons for pursuing the same strategy:

If I have HIV I can just go out and spread it to 100 people so that we all go together. Why should they be left behind having fun if I must die? (ibid.)

Leclerc-Madlala argues as follows:

By spreading the virus one is sharing the burden, the anger, the hopelessness and ultimately the death. It is no longer an individual problem but a shared group problem ... If you think you have got it, spread it. This seems to be the predominant ideology shaping the sexual activities of young people in the HIV/AIDS epidemic. For better or for worse, many of KwaZulu-Natal's urban dwelling youth have developed an acute sense of group destiny. They share a philosophy which says 'If I don't have a future (now because of AIDS), then I will try my best to ensure that others don't have one either'. In the words of one 19-year-old female student: 'by giving it to others, I won't be going down alone. That's my only hope. That's my comfort. It's as simple as that' (ibid. 371).

Under these circumstances, it is possible to construct a plausible hypothesis that by providing the hope of a longer life through HAART, inroads can be made into this destructive sexual cultural response. (Such an hypothesis is at least as plausible as the assumption that the increase in risk behaviour among some MSM in the advanced capitalist countries is a result of HAART.) It is a reasonable proposition that a social response to AIDS that includes treatment – and thus the gift of hope and longer life for those already infected – is likely to deliver greater social benefits (in terms of lower rates of HIV transmission) than an uncaring response that effectively consigns a large cohort of young people to the dustbin of history. At the very least, it will encourage people to come forward for testing. As one young man said, 'If you know (that you are HIV-positive), that does not help because you are still going to die anyway, because there is no treatment for the disease. So I don't approve of taking the test' (cited in Mapolisa 2001: 47). Offering the hope of treatment is likely to encourage more people with views such as these to participate in VCT. There is evidence that fear of a positive test result is a major barrier to participation in VCT in South Africa (Ginwalla *et al.* 2002). The possibility of accessing HAART if the test proves positive could thus help break down this barrier.

Of course hopelessness is not simply a product of AIDS. High unemployment, particularly among the youth (see Table 4.8), no doubt also contributes to a jaundiced view of the future. According to a survey of adults in Khayelitsha-Mitchell's Plain (working class areas of Cape Town), 72% of the unemployed either agreed, or agreed strongly with the statement: 'I feel useless and depressed because I do not have a job.'[2] If it is the case that social marginalisation is fostered by HIV infection and unemployment, then providing HAART is only one arm of the necessary intervention. Providing hope through job creation and poverty relief must be an integrated part of the response. This issue is touched upon in Chapter 7.

Combating myths about AIDS

Another way in which the failure to provide HAART could lead to an increase in high-risk behaviour has to do with myths about curing AIDS. In the absence of a national treatment programme, it is possible that more people will latch onto myths about AIDS cures. Some of these are harmless (such as 'the African potato cures AIDS'[3]) but others, particularly the myth that 'having sex with a virgin cures AIDS', contribute to the spread of HIV.

The myth that sex with a virgin can help 'clean the blood' is common in other parts of Africa and is similar to the belief in nineteenth-century England that sex with a child could cure syphilis (Leclerc-Madlala 1997: 375). It has been linked to the reported increase in child rape and the sharp increase in HIV-infection among young girls (ibid.). However, it is unclear how widespread this myth is. According to a recent national household study, 88% of respondents disagreed with the statement 'AIDS can be cured by sex with a virgin', 10% said they didn't know, and 2% agreed (Shisana and Simbayi 2002: 82). This survey, however, probably undersampled high-risk groups – such as those living in informal settlements, in hostels and in the army. The proportion of people who believe this myth (or who think it might be true) may well be higher. A study of young South Africans found that 7% of respondents agreed with the statement 'Having sex with a virgin cures you of AIDS' and 18% said they did not know (LoveLife 2000: 23). According to a study of truck drivers in 1999, 35% thought that sex with a virgin would protect them from or cure them of AIDS (Marcus 2001: 116). As truck drivers are particularly at risk of contracting HIV, their adherence to this myth is particularly worrying.

A large-scale national prevention and treatment programme can help combat such myths by improving information about AIDS and by demonstrating that HAART offers the chance of a longer, better-quality life for those living with AIDS. One can reasonably hypothesise that as more people respond to antiretroviral treatment, explanations and actions based on medical science rather than mythology will gain credence.

HAART and stigma

Another way in which HAART has the potential to reduce risky sexual behaviour is by encouraging disclosure of HIV status and reducing the general level of stigmatisation of people living with AIDS. This has been the experience of pilot HAART projects in Khayelitsha (Coetzee and Boulle 2003) and in Botswana (Ramotlhwa 2003). Evidence such as this suggest that these social effects are important and could contribute substantially to creating a social environment less conducive to HIV transmission. The ASSA2000 Interventions Model does not allow for these effects, and in this regard is probably underestimating the impact of HAART on prevention.

The stigmatisation of people with AIDS contributes to their pain and suffering, and increases the social and economic vulnerability of those (particularly young people) living in AIDS-affected African households (Strode and Grant 2001). The stigmatisation of AIDS is also a 'powerful, pernicious force that is an important barrier to prevention efforts' (De Cock *et al.* 2002: 69). To the extent that HAART reduces stigma, it thus contributes to prevention. According to Galvao, there are important social benefits associated with the Brazilian government's policy of providing free access to HAART for people living with AIDS. She highlights the

social recognition gained when the government defended their rights to treatment, and thereby their value and importance to society as a whole. In this respect, the distribution programme has helped to avert what one Brazilian activist called – in less favourable times – the 'civil death' of people living with HIV/AIDS (2002: 1863).

Providing access to treatment for AIDS sufferers can also help address stigma by encouraging people to disclose their HIV-status. According to Farmer *et al.*, a HAART programme in rural Haiti has contributed to a shift in social attitudes:

Although AIDS remains a stigmatised disease in Haiti, we believe that access to effective therapy has lessened AIDS-related stigma. The demand for HIV testing and the opportunity of counselling has risen since HAART was made available (2001: 405).

This particular HAART intervention entailed directly observed therapy (DOT) whereby each HIV patient was assigned an 'accompagnateur' (usually a community health worker) to observe the ingestion of pills, to respond to patient and family concerns, and to offer moral support (ibid.). This DOT-HAART programme thus clearly entails disclosure of the HAART patient to his or her family, and probably also the wider community. This is what gives the intervention its transformative properties: greater disclosure means less secrecy and less stigmatisation born out of ignorance and fear.

But this very transformative aspect of the programme may be problematic in the sense that it encourages (perhaps forces?) people to disclose their HIV status when they otherwise would choose not to do so. As Pawinski *et al.* argue: 'The issue of confidentiality requires serious consideration in a DOT-HAART programme, since many patients might want status to remain confidential from family, friends, neighbours, shopkeepers and community health-care workers' (2002: 624). They go on to cite evidence from KwaZulu-Natal that many HIV-positive people prefer not to disclose their HIV status (ibid.). Fear of disclosure and lack of confidentiality has also been implicated as a barrier to participation in VCT in Africa (e.g. Pool *et al.* 2002; Ginwalla *et al.* 2002).

De Cock *et al.* (2002) argue that one of the reasons why the AIDS pandemic has gained such a grip in Africa is that the public health response has not sought to challenge this 'quest for secrecy' more effectively. Ramotlhwa (2003) makes a similar point with regard to Botswana, arguing that the 'confidentiality paradigm' has prioritised human rights concerns over public health issues and that routine HIV testing should be introduced. A well-designed DOT-HAART intervention could contribute to such transformation of attitudes. In cases where social attitudes are strongly negative towards HIV-positive people, greater preparation work is required – such as community-level education programmes and stronger support facilities for those on HAART. Negative social attitudes towards people with AIDS should not be a reason for inaction – instead, appropriate policies should be designed to address them. In the case of the rural Haiti study, the process of training the 'accompagnateur' to provide the necessary support to people on HAART would itself have contributed to improving community-level information about the needs of, and social and personal challenges faced by, people living with AIDS.

Clearly, a DOT-HAART programme is more intensive of resources than a HAART programme, because community health workers would need to be trained and mobilised. This will add to the cost of the programme. However, as this results in better adherence to the therapy (and hence less resistance and superior health outcomes) and has the potential to contribute to attitude shifts at the community level, it is very likely that the additional expenditure would pay for itself in terms of lower morbidity and (potentially) lower rates of HIV transmission. However, as there is no data on this effect, it is difficult to include it in a model such as the ASSA2000 Interventions Model.

It is, however, important to note that a HAART programme that does not entail DOT is still capable of fighting stigma. This is because the very existence of a treatment programme is likely to facilitate greater openness and dialogue about AIDS. Brian Brink, the director of Anglo American's AIDS policy, has reported that the company's decision to provide HAART to its HIV-positive workers resulted in 'a complete transformation in attitude', with patients being far more willing to talk about AIDS.[4]

5.3 Voluntary counselling and testing and behaviour change

The ASSA2000 Interventions Model does not allow for any increase or decrease in sexual risk behaviour as a result of the introduction of HAART per se, although it does assume that the accompanying VCT causes behaviour change. Is this a valid assumption? Can we assume that VCT is likely to encourage safer sex? On the basis of recent South African household survey data, Shisana and Simbayi argued that there is evidence that VCT leads to safer sexual practices:

When adults who had had an HIV test were compared to those who had not done so, it was found that 25.1% of the former (n=1,659) used a condom at last sex as compared to 20.2% of the latter (n=5,364). This suggests that HIV testing has a positive influence on condom use (2002: 76).

While a strong case can be made that HIV testing and counselling is *likely* to promote behaviour change, one cannot read the direction of causality from simple correlation (as done above). Quantitative household survey data of this kind need to be supplemented with information from randomised trials, and by more qualitative information about the relationship between VCT and behaviour change.

The central difficulty with generalising from non-experimental studies of the impact of VCT is that there is an inherent selection bias in these studies: those who voluntarily choose to undergo VCT are not likely to be random. They probably have reason to be concerned about their past sexual behaviour and are informed sufficiently about AIDS to be concerned about their possible HIV status. This makes it very difficult to draw conclusions about causation from empirical information about the relationship between VCT and HIV status or sexual behaviour.

One of the sources of information used by the demographers who designed the ASSA2000 Interventions Model was a randomised trial in Kenya, Tanzania and Trinidad (VCTESG 2000). The study was set up explicitly to determine the efficacy of VCT in reducing unprotected sexual intercourse among individuals and sex-partner couples in Nairobi, Dar es Salaam and Port of Spain. Individuals and couples were randomly assigned VCT or basic health information. At the first follow-up (between three and seven months after the base-line), those who had been provided with basic health information were offered VCT, and those who had been offered VCT were offered retesting. A second follow-up asked questions about sexual behaviour.

This study is important for two reasons: it took place in developing countries (two of which were in Africa); and it was a randomised trial. The study found that

the proportion of individuals reporting unprotected intercourse with non-primary partners declined significantly more for those receiving VCT than those receiving health information (men, 35% reduction with VCT versus 13% reduction with health information; women, 39% reduction with VCT versus 17% reduction with health information) (VCTESG 2000: 103).

This represents strong support for the proposition that VCT affects behaviour change.

Note that this study compared two interventions (VCT versus providing basic health information). It did not compare VCT with the 'do nothing' scenario (as this would have been unethical). If it had, then the benefits in terms of behaviour change would almost certainly have been greater. This is because providing some basic health information probably also affects behaviour – although the evidence concerning the link between information about AIDS and behaviour change is not strong.

Sweat *et al.* (2000), in their study of the cost-effectiveness of VCT in Kenya and Tanzania, found that the intervention did lead to behaviour change, and that it was most cost-effective with regard to HIV-positive people and for those who received VCT as a couple. Other studies have also found that counselling couples had major benefits in terms of facilitating disclosure and negotiating risk reduction strategies (VCTESG 2000: 109–10). According to De Cock *et al.*, 'increased efforts are required to arrange for couples to be tested together for HIV infection, so that HIV/AIDS can be approached as a disease of the family and of society' (2002: 70).

The argument that AIDS should be treated as 'a disease of the family and of society' is an important one. One of the limitations of using counselling as a tool to facilitate behaviour change is that it concentrates on the individual rather than the social context within which that individual behaves. As pointed out in Chapter 1, there are strong socio-economic determinants of HIV transmission (see Figure 1.3). Providing people with information and advice may not be sufficient to bring about lower rates of HIV transmission. Sexual culture and relationship dynamics often prevent the translation of information into sexual behaviour change.

The challenge posed by sexual culture

Sexual cultures comprise the age-specific and collectively developed beliefs, expectations and rules for sexual conduct that 'govern the sorts of activities defined as legitimate and how sexual encounters are to be staged' (Crothers 2001: 12). Leclerc-Madlala argues that the sexual culture in parts of KwaZulu-Natal is 'underpinned by meanings which associate sex with gifts, and manliness with the ability to attract and maintain multiple sexual partners' (2002: 31–2). Such sexual cultures clearly contribute to the spread of HIV and need to be addressed as part of any intervention to promote behaviour change.

But this is a difficult task because sexual cultures are socially constructed and reflect unequal gender relations in the broader society. Leclerc-Madlala's ethnographic work describes Zulu sexual culture as characterised by

gender inequity, transactional sex, the socio-cultural *isoka* ideal of multiple sexual part-nerships, lack of discussion on matters of sexuality in the home and between sexual partners, the conditioning of both men and women to accept sexual violence as 'normal' masculine behaviour along with the 'right' of men to control sexual encounters, and the existence of increasingly discordant and contested gender scripts (2001: 41).

Similar findings were reported by Harrison *et al.* (2001) in their study of adolescents in rural KwaZulu-Natal, and by Mapolisa (2001) in his study of young African men in Cape Town. Leclerc-Madlala argues that it is these characteristics, together with social pressure to prove fertility,[5] which creates a 'socio-sexual culture/context that makes behaviour change such a difficulty' (2002: 29).

Note that risky sexual culture is not limited to the African population in South Africa. According to a qualitative study of white university students, multiple partnering (both serial and concurrent) is usual, as is the pursuit of casual sex for its own sake (Marcus 2002: 32). Marcus comments that although 'white students perceive themselves to be very different from their black colleagues, the sexual social environment they describe does not appear to differ in qualitative terms, at least in terms of serial and concurrent multiple partnering' (ibid.).

Counselling people in couples can help facilitate critical discussion about the particular sexual culture they are part of, and help bring about behaviour change. This is particularly important in sexual cultures where there is a high level of violence against women – such as is the case in South Africa.[6] There is clearly a need to address the endemic problem of violence against women both through better law enforcement and interventions at community level to combat sexual sub-cultures where rape is considered to be a normal, recreational activity (Wojcicki 2002). However, given the high level of sexual coercion within relationships[7] (Eaton *et al.* 2003: 161), there is also a role for bringing about improved sexual relationships through counselling people in couples.

Sexual cultures characterised by high-risk behaviour pose challenges for behavioural interventions. Consequently, intervention strategies need to be carefully and innovatively designed so that they are meaningful to the participants. For example, a participatory workshop programme in the Gambia was successful because it focussed on infertility prevention rather than family planning (i.e. was not seen as promoting unwelcome values) and included men:

The infertility prevention approach, rather than a focus on HIV or family planning, means that the programme responded to issues deemed important by men. This made it possible at the start to obtain permission to discuss sexual health issues, a topic which normally intimidates extension workers. Later, the men became convinced that poor relations with their partners could put them at risk of infection, and therefore that increased trust between themselves and their wives was in their self-interest (Paine *et al.* 2002: 47).

Another innovative and community-based intervention was that in Carltonville, a mining town in South Africa. The intervention reached out to migrant workers, sex workers and members of the broader community (Williams *et al.* 2000).

Sexual cultures are far from immutable. As described above, there are indications that sexual culture among young Zulu speakers has responded to the AIDS pandemic in ways that contribute to the spread of AIDS. However, not all sexual cultural change has been harmful. According to focus group research among Zulu-speaking male adolescents, most young men believed *isoka* (the practice of multiple sexual partnerships) was risky and stupid (Tillotson and Maharaj 2001: 95). There is also evidence that in South African sentinel sites where there is high media penetration, self-perpetuating cultures of risk-prevention (such as increased condom use among non-cohabiting youth) are taking shape (Kelly, cited in Leclerc-Madlala 2002: 25). A recent survey of young South Africans found that only a fifth of those already sexually active participated in sex for money arrangements (LoveLife 2000: 18) – but there were still worryingly high reported rates of sexual coercion (ibid. 19).

These indications of changing sexual cultures suggest that there is space for VCT to help facilitate behaviour change. And, given that high levels of AIDS information in South Africa do not seem to translate into an equivalent concern to adopt safe sexual practices,[8] there is clearly a need to supplement AIDS information campaigns with VCT interventions. VCT can help reinforce AIDS education while probing the individual social and psychological circumstances that may make behaviour change difficult. In their review of South African AIDS counselling services, Richter *et al.* note that VCT is 'a demonstrably effective secondary prevention strategy whereby HIV-positive individuals reduce their risk of infecting others and of themselves being reinfected' (2001: 152), but go on to argue that for VCT programmes to be effective, they need to be part of a 'circle of care which links both HIV-positive and HIV-negative people to a comprehensive set of services after HIV testing' (ibid. 153). They particularly stress the importance of providing additional services to support the poverty-related needs of those participating in AIDS counselling programmes.

The link between poverty and sexual behaviour (see Chapter 1) poses major challenges for AIDS interventions. To the extent that women's sexual behaviour is a product of economic circumstances, interventions at the level of individual behaviour and sexual culture are unlikely to be very successful. Leclerc-Madlala found in her study of young Zulu women that promiscuity and transactional sex were in part a product of the post-apartheid political economy:

> For most, the present economic situation seems to be a major driving force in their new sexual assertiveness. It was apparent from my field work experience that many young women 'played the field' for all it was worth, and the 'worth' was definitely calculated in financial terms ... Some women claimed that their parents encouraged multiple relationships both directly and indirectly, as it ensured an additional flow of money into the household (2001: 43–4).

Other studies also point to the prevalence of transactional sex, highlighting the dangers of sexual violence that face those engaging in 'survivalist sex' (Wojcicki 2002).

Given these conditions, it is clear that addressing poverty has to be a major component of any strategy to combat HIV/AIDS effectively. South Africa's high levels of poverty and inequality pose specific challenges for the way the country deals with the 'development dilemma'. The final two chapters consider this issue. Chapter 6 argues that the impact of AIDS on economic growth has unsettling implications for income distribution and Chapter 7 argues that AIDS and poverty should be addressed together.

6 AIDS, economic growth and inequality in South Africa

As discussed in Chapter 1, the AIDS pandemic is both a cause and effect of poverty. Poverty, in turn, is a function of low levels of economic development and high inequality. The relationship between AIDS, economic growth and income distribution is thus central to the development dilemma posed by AIDS. This chapter reviews the existing macroeconomic modelling work on the impact of AIDS on economic growth in South Africa and poses the question of the likely impact of AIDS on inequality.

Figure 1.4 in Chapter 1 outlined some of the ways in which the AIDS pandemic reduces economic growth – thus increasing poverty (and exacerbating the risks of HIV infection). Chapters 3 and 4 opened the discussion of the economic cost of AIDS by exploring the costs and benefits of various AIDS interventions (including treatment) in South Africa. With regard to MTCTP, it was argued that the government would save money by acting to save children from HIV infection. Providing HAART to adults, by contrast, would save lives, but the costs in terms of the government budget are likely to be substantial.

What has been missing from the discussion so far, however, has been any explicit consideration of the inter-relationship between poverty, AIDS and economic growth. Despite highlighting this issue in the opening chapter, the demographic modelling work used in Chapters 3 and 4 (the ASSA2000 Interventions Model) took no cognisance of the impact of the growth path on the pandemic, or of the impact of the pandemic on economic growth. It would, of course, be unreasonable to expect demographic models to capture the complex interplay of AIDS and growth as sketched in Figures 1.3 and 1.4 in Chapter 1. But this does not mean that economic dynamics can safely be assumed away. Rather, it is important to understand how AIDS affects growth in South Africa, how businesses are responding to the pandemic, and the likely impact on inequality and poverty. This is the task undertaken in this chapter.

6.1 Some relevant demographics

Macroeconomic models of the impact of AIDS make extensive use of available demographic research on the impact of AIDS on different parts of the labour force. But this information is often uneven and contradictory. For example, a 2002 national survey concluded that there are no significant differences in HIV prevalence between the employed and the unemployed

(Shisana and Simbayi 2002: 53). There are, however, problems of bias regarding the HIV-prevalence data in this survey.[1] Most demographic modelling indicates that HIV-prevalence rates are 30–50% higher among the unemployed, largely because of the large share of young, female African people (BER 2000: 7).

HIV prevalence appears to vary between skill levels. According to a recent firm-based survey in Swaziland, employees in the lowest income band had the highest HIV prevalence (42.6%), followed by 32.4% in the next band, 28.9% in the higher-skilled band, and 13.4% in the highest-skilled and professional band (Evian 2003: 7). These differences were all statistically significant, whereas HIV prevalence between age bands was not (see Table 1.2, Chapter 1). Drawing on insurance data and other private-sector information, Dorrington (2001) reports that South Africans in the higher job grades have an HIV prevalence of only 2.5% to 3%.[2] This information was used in the ASSA2000 model to fit the epidemic curves for white and Asian people (who tend to be concentrated in the higher job grades), rather than the antenatal survey data (which is unreliable for higher-income groups). The ASSA2000 model predicts that population HIV prevalence will peak at 3.2% (2011) for whites,[3] at 4.8% (2010) for Asians, at 6% (2010) for 'coloureds' (i.e. mixed race) and at 19.5% (2006) for Africans.

One of the problems with the demographic models for economic analysis is the difficulty involved in teasing out the impact of race from other variables such as skills and income. As noted above, the ASSA2000 model used information on HIV prevalence by skill to project epidemic curves for whites and Asians. However, for Africans and coloureds, researchers have had to move from information about race to assumptions about HIV prevalence by skill category. The Metropolitan and ING-Barings macro-economic models (discussed below) derive HIV skills profiles by 'overlaying' the 1996 census data on occupation with age, gender and racial HIV profiles per province (ING-Barings 2000: 7). This results in a far higher estimate for HIV prevalence among skilled workers in 2000 (7.2% for highly skilled workers, to 12.1% for skilled workers and 14.3% for unskilled workers) than is assumed in the ASSA2000 model.

These highly varying estimates of prevalence by skill level are a problem for macroeconomic modellers because of the profound impact of skills shortages on economic growth. As can be seen in Table 6.1, unemployment among the highly skilled is already very low. According to an ILO study, more than 60% of South African firms in 2000 reported that they would have problems replacing skilled labour (ILO 2000: 5). The

point at which the economy 'runs out' of skilled labour has major implications for the projected macroeconomic impact of AIDS. According to
the Metropolitan model, 1.4% of highly skilled workers will have full-blown
AIDS by 2005, this estimate rising to 3.5% in 2015 (ABT/Metropolitan
2000). Given that less than 1% of the highly skilled are unemployed, there
will not be nearly enough people to replace those dying of AIDS in these
categories. The steady drain of skilled professionals (Meyer *et al.* 2000) as
a result of emigration is no doubt exacerbating the situation. Therefore,
unless firms react by providing their skilled workers with life-prolonging
HAART, the economy will be constrained by skills shortages and skilled
wage pressure (as described in BER 2001). This constraint will kick in later
if the ASSA2000 estimates are closer to the mark.

Table 6.1 *The structure of South Africa's labour force (1996 census)*

	Highly skilled***		Skilled**		Semi- & unskilled*	
Economically active	Number	%	Number	%	Number	%
Formally employed	1,300,009	92.1	2,899,334	76.5	3,509,890	40.9
Informally employed	100,177	7.1	289,901	7.7	710,223	8.3
Unemployed	11,148	0.8	598,083	15.8	4,366,238	50.8
Total labour force	1,411,334	100	3,787,318	100	8,586,351	100
Composition (%)	10.2%		27.5%		62.3%	
HIV prevalence in 2005 (2015)#	13.3% (18.3%)		20.2% (25.4%)		22.8% (27.6%)	
AIDS prevalence in 2005 (2015)#	1.4% (3.5%)		1.9% (4.2%)		2.2% (4.7%)	

Source: BER 2001: 11, 12. *** Highly skilled (professional, semi-professional and
technical occupations; managerial, administrative and executive occupations).
** Skilled (clerical services and sales occupations; farmers, farm managers,
artisans, apprentices and related occupations; production foreman, production
adviser). * Semi-skilled and unskilled (all occupations not defined as highly
skilled or skilled). # Data from ABT/Metropolitan.

The close association between unemployment and poverty in South Africa
has been well established (see Chapter 4, Section 4.4). A household survey
in the Free State province indicates that AIDS-affected households are in a
particularly vulnerable position, having higher rates of unemployment

and being more dependent on non-employment income like pensions (Booysen *et al.* 2001; Booysen 2002b). This suggests that one or more of the following is the case: people living in households with limited (if any) access to wage employment are more vulnerable to HIV infection; that AIDS-affected households have experienced disproportionate employment losses because of AIDS; and that people living with AIDS migrate to households with pensioners in order to be taken care of (or that pensioners move to households where there are people sick with AIDS).

What does this mean for overall inequality? All else being equal, households that lose a breadwinner through AIDS will become poorer and shift down the income distribution. If the job is taken by a previously unemployed person, then that person's household income will rise and the household will move up the income distribution. The overall Gini coefficient will thus remain broadly unchanged. However, if firms react by cutting back on the number of jobs, then the number of households without access to a breadwinner will rise, thus worsening the Gini coefficient. If average wages rise at the same time (perhaps in response to increased pressure from workers to compensate them for the burden of higher medical insurance and health expenditure, or perhaps because the average worker is becoming more skilled as firms get rid of unskilled workers first) then inequality will worsen further.

At this point the importance of economic modelling becomes clear. Questions such as 'what is the likely impact of AIDS on labour demand and income' need to be answered before anything can be said about the impact of AIDS on income distribution. But the issue goes beyond the partial equilibrium impact of labour demand and wages. We need to know how the impact of AIDS on firms (and the government) feeds through the economy to impact on the level of national income.

Any discussion of the impact of AIDS on distribution requires information about the size of the pie (the GDP) and the number of people in need of a slice (the population). AIDS slows income growth – but it also slows population growth. If the population falls faster than income, then per capita income will rise. But while this is theoretically possible, it is not common. Econometric research indicates that AIDS has either had an insignificant impact on the growth of per capita income in developing countries (Bloom and Mahal 1997) or has reduced it (Bonnel 2000).[4] Bonnel's results indicate that 'in the case of a typical sub-Saharan country with a prevalence rate of 20%', the growth rate of per capita income would be reduced by 1.2 percentage points a year because of AIDS (ibid. 846). But whether absolute per capita income is higher or lower as a result of AIDS in any particular country is ultimately an empirical question.

As shown below, two of the three substantial South African models predict a rise in per capita income, whereas the third predicts a fall.[5] Whether per capita income rises or falls has disturbing ethical and policy implications. The Malthusian possibility that AIDS may increase per capita income might suggest to those policy makers with no respect for human life that AIDS may in some sense be 'welfare-enhancing'. They may conclude that it is economically rational to do little to prevent the AIDS pandemic from taking its course. Leaving aside the moral and ethical problems of such a position, it does point to the importance of producing the best possible macroeconomic modelling work and showing how different assumptions and theoretical underpinnings produce different results.

6.2 Modelling the macroeconomic impact of AIDS

This section provides a critical overview of recent macroeconomic research on the impact of AIDS in South Africa. It is not a comprehensive bibliographic review (as in CADRE 2000a and 2000b), but rather a selective analysis of recent and important pieces of economic research. The key objective is to explain in an accessible manner how different macro-economic models arrive at different results and to point to the limitations of these models – in particular, their failure to take into account the dynamic adjustments suggested by firm-level studies. See also Van den Heever (2003) and Booysen et al. (2003) for reviews of South African macro-economic models.

The earliest attempts to model the economic impact of AIDS in South Africa were those of Broomberg et al. (1991) and Trotter (1993). They adopted a 'human capital' approach that summed up both the expected direct costs of AIDS (i.e. health costs) as well as indirect costs (discounted lost future earnings) over time. However, such approaches do not consider the full macroeconomic ramifications of these costs on the rate and pattern of economic growth.

Macroeconomic modelling of the impact of AIDS typically entails three steps. First, the modellers use an existing macroeconomic model to project what growth would look like in the absence of AIDS. Then they hypothesise a set of 'channels' through which the pandemic is assumed to affect the broader economy. Finally, they estimate (and guesstimate) the size of these various effects, plug the assumptions into the model and see what growth path results. This 'growth with AIDS' scenario is then con-trasted with the 'growth without AIDS' scenario.

A major limitation of this approach is, of course, the assumption that the current growth path is the 'growth in the absence of AIDS'. While this was a reasonable assumption for models in the late 1980s and even early 1990s, it is becoming increasingly problematic. As McPherson *et al.* put it, the impact of AIDS cannot

be treated as an 'exogenous' influence that can be 'tacked on' to models derived on the presumption that the workforce is HIV-free. HIV/AIDS has become an 'endogenous' influence on most African countries that has adversely affected their potential for growth and development (2000: 3).

This is particularly the case in South Africa. Employment has fallen so sharply over the past decade that Fedderke and Mariotti (2002) argue that a 'structural break' took place in 1990. While a range of factors (including labour market regulation and globalisation) contributed to this, it is also very likely that firms have been reacting to the presence, and threat, of AIDS in the workforce by shedding jobs – particularly among the unskilled.[6] If the impact of AIDS is already being felt in the 'no-AIDS' scenarios, then either the impact of AIDS will be underestimated in the subsequent comparative analysis, and/or the modelling of economic dynamics will be compromised.

It is also worth emphasising that the estimated impact depends largely on the nature and design of the macroeconomic model. The first big modelling exercise (ING-Barings 2000) used time series information together with a social accounting matrix (SAM) that provided more detailed household-level data. Arndt and Lewis (2000) made use of the same SAM, but in the context of a more neoclassical computational general equilibrium (CGE) model. The most recent macroeconomic modelling exercise – that of the Bureau for Economic Research at Stellenbosch University (BER 2001) – does not use a SAM, but instead builds on their Keynesian framework using insights from available research, including that by ING-Barings.

There are many 'channels' through which the AIDS pandemic can affect the broader economy. AIDS has an immediate (or 'first order') impact on the size (and efficiency) of the labour force. But while demographic models can provide a broad indication of the impact of AIDS on the size of the labour force, the impact on the efficiency of the labour force is much harder to estimate. As noted above, there is still relatively little data on the distribution of HIV prevalence across skill bands – although recent evidence from Swaziland indicates a clear and significant negative relationship between skill level and HIV prevalence (see above).

The other first-order impact of AIDS is on pattern of consumption (i.e. it is typically assumed that more household resources will be allocated to health care[7]). Although there is an emerging body of household-level research (e.g. Booysen et al. 2001; Booysen 2002b; Johnson et al. 2002), there is as yet no information that can be generalised to the national level. Methodological problems concerning the drawing of samples and the definition of AIDS-affected households make it difficult to compare the results of (and generalise from) the existing studies of the economic impact of AIDS on households (Dike 2002).

Studies from South Africa and other developing countries are suggestive, but often contradictory. For example, there is research showing that households may erode savings by paying for the health costs of AIDS sufferers – or they may increase savings in order to support surviving household members (see Ainsworth & Over 1994; and CADRE 2000a). Given that HIV infection is concentrated among poorer South Africans, it is unlikely that savings will increase as a result of AIDS. Booysen et al. (2001) found that AIDS-affected households draw on available savings to finance medical costs and funerals, but Samson (2002a)[8] found an indeterminate impact of AIDS on household savings. Oni et al. (2002) concluded that AIDS-affected households had lower levels of savings and higher levels of borrowing from relatives than households not affected by AIDS. According to Booysen (2002b), AIDS-affected households in QwaQwa borrowed money from friends and relatives, whereas those in Welkom were more likely to borrow from micro-lenders. Higher borrowing from relatives probably translates into lower levels of savings by these relatives, and borrowing from micro-lenders almost certainly results in AIDS-affected households being caught in a debt trap. In short, studies of savings behaviour remain limited to isolated household studies and there is as yet no reliable estimate of the overall impact of AIDS on total household savings.

Research in Africa indicates that AIDS-affected households shift spending away from durable goods and towards non-durables (ILO 2000: 5–7; ABT Associates 2000: 52; Desmond et al. 2000; Booysen et al. 2001). This does not, however, mean that the overall pattern of demand will change in this direction. Firstly, AIDS-affected households could spend relatively less on durables *and* absolutely less on non-durables like food. In such a scenario, the demand for both durables and non-durables will fall. Secondly, the overall impact on the pattern of consumption is mediated by the distribution of AIDS-affected households across the income distribution (and by differential consumption patterns across income brackets).

For example, the ING-Barings model assumes that AIDS will result in a greater share of income going to richer households (as skilled wages rise in response to skilled labour shortages). Data in the SAM used by ING-Barings indicate that richer households spend more on services and durable goods than do poorer households. Thus as skilled workers rise up the income distribution, the model predicts that this will cushion the impact (to some extent) of lower demand for durable goods from AIDS-affected households.[9] The ING-Barings model uses demographic data on the expected size of the labour force and then 'weights' it to account for skill composition (i.e. skilled labour carries a higher weight) and adjusts it downwards to account for loss of productivity as a result of AIDS.[10] This has been criticised by CADRE (2000b: 14) on the grounds that it probably underestimates the contribution to productivity of experienced workers in lower-skill categories (and hence underestimates the costs of replacing such workers), and underestimates the potential for high-skill capacity bottlenecks in some sectors.

AIDS also affects people indirectly – i.e. through the impact of 'second-order' effects that occur after firms and the government have responded to the first-order impact of AIDS. These impacts are even more difficult to estimate, and will vary according to economic sector, degree of competition, market structure, etc. In the case of relatively competitive markets, does one assume that firms will respond to higher medical costs for employees and lower productivity by replacing labour with machinery – and if so, by how much? And, will the firms respond to higher (direct and indirect) labour costs by raising prices (i.e. passing costs on to consumers) or reducing profits (thereby probably reducing investment in subsequent periods)? To what extent will they share the costs with workers by constraining wage growth, thereby lowering consumer demand and growth in subsequent periods? The different models assume different scenarios, and model the way in which the assumptions impact on economic growth in different ways.[11]

There are similar problems regarding the reaction of the government to the AIDS pandemic. Will the government increase spending on health – and if so, will this be at the cost of lower spending on other items; and if so which? Whether cuts are made to military or education expenditure has very different implications for long-run growth. Alternatively, one could assume that the government responds by increasing borrowing or taxation to finance the increase in health spending. Depending on the nature of the macroeconomic model, such increases have further knock-on effects. In more Keynesian models (like ING-Barings and BER) deficit-financed health spending increases demand and growth, whereas in the CGE model of Arndt and Lewis, increased borrowing reduces private investment and hence constrains growth over time.

The ING-Barings and BER models

Both the ING-Barings and BER models predict a slight worsening of the ratio of budget deficit to GDP as the government faces the dual pressure of depressed tax revenues and increased demand for spending on health. They assume that the government will continue on the path of fiscal discipline and not engage in excessive borrowing or inflationary forms of financing the deficit. However, the BER model assumes greater wage pressure as a result of AIDS (driven primarily by skilled-labour shortages) and assumes that the Reserve Bank responds to such inflationary forces by pushing up interest rates.

Despite these differences, the ING-Barings and BER models arrive at broadly similar findings with regard to GDP and employment (see Table 6.2). They both estimate that AIDS will reduce the growth rate of GDP by 0.6 percentage points per annum. As AIDS is assumed to reduce population growth by more than it reduces GDP growth, both models predict an increase in per capita income (of just under one percentage point per annum). A similar logic underpins the prediction in both models that the rate of unemployment will fall as a result of the AIDS pandemic (employment falls, but because the labour force falls faster, the proportion of those without work decreases relative to that which would have occurred in a no-AIDS scenario).

Despite similarities in the overall growth impact, the BER and ING-Barings models tell different stories as to why growth is constrained by AIDS. Whereas the ING-Barings model assumes that lower labour supply and lower labour productivity will induce firms to invest in capital equipment (thus preventing investment demand from falling in the aggregate),[12] the BER model assumes that investment will be limited by shortages of skilled workers (needed to operate the capital equipment) and by reduced profitability. ING-Barings tells the story of a 'vicious cycle' in which reduced household income translates into lower consumption spending – which translates into lower demand and hence lower growth and household income. By contrast, the BER model assumes that there will be a strong upward pressure on skilled wages (as skills shortages intensify and as workers resist the erosion of their take-home pay as a result of the rising costs of medical insurance). The BER modellers assume that the increase in wages will exceed any decrease in employment – and thus that wage increases will boost household income in the aggregate (although by implication it will be more concentrated in the hands of those households that still have employed members).

Table 6.2 *Percentage point differences between the AIDS and no-AIDS scenarios in the ING-Barings (2000) and Bureau for Economic Research (2001) macroeconomic models*

Impact of AIDS on:	ING-Barings (2000) 2002–2015	BER (2001) 2002–2015
Real GDP growth p.a.	−0.6	−0.5
Real gross domestic fixed investment growth p.a.	0.0	−1.2
Real private consumption growth p.a.	−0.7	−0.3
Total population growth p.a.**	−1.5	−1.3
Total labour force growth p.a.***	−1.2	−1.6
Employment growth p.a.****	−0.6	−0.6
Growth in the unemployment rate (i.e. % of labour force without formal jobs)*	−0.9	−2
Real per capita GDP growth p.a.#	0.9	0.9
Interest rate (% point difference in the level)	0.6	2.9
Budget deficit/GDP (% point difference in the level)	0.7	0.2

* Figures for BER estimated from level data in 2001: 38. ** Figures for ING-Barings calculated from data in 2000: 6. *** Figures for ING-Barings calculated from data in 2000: 10. NB data for ING-Barings is a labour force figure weighted by skill level. **** Employment figure for ING-Barings estimated from data in 2000: 2. # Figures for ING-Barings calculated from data in the table.

Neither model provides an explicit projection for income distribution, although both predict that the share of income going to higher-income households will rise over time (ING-Barings 2000: 14; BER 2001: 31–2). But at the same time, the models predict that average living standards (i.e. per capita income) will rise relative to a no-AIDS scenario and that one of the central determinants of poverty, unemployment, will fall.

The Arndt and Lewis model

The macroeconomic model of Arndt and Lewis (2000) contains different assumptions and arrives at different conclusions. Arndt and Lewis assume a far greater negative impact on productivity and investment, and a far greater impact on government spending and interest rates.[13] Largely as a result of this, they project a much greater impact on GDP growth – i.e. growth is reduced by an average of about two percentage points a year between 2002 and 2010. They attribute almost half (45%) the blame for this to the increase in the government deficit (which in their model 'crowds out' private investment) and about a third (34%) of the blame to the negative impact of AIDS on total factor productivity growth (2000: 879–81).

This drop in growth is sufficiently large to exceed the drop in population – and hence per capita income in their model is projected to fall. They conclude that per capita income in 2010 will be 8% lower than it would otherwise have been in the absence of the AIDS pandemic (ibid. 877). Arndt and Lewis show that if government-related AIDS expenditures and private expenditure on health and food is excluded, then per capita income declines by 13% (relative to the no-AIDS scenario). They thus conclude that 'the survivors of the AIDS epidemic are left with a smaller economic "pie" and more of this pie is directed towards non-discretionary health and food expenditures' (ibid.).

Also, unlike the BER and ING-Barings models, Arndt and Lewis predict that the unemployment rate among semi-skilled and unskilled workers will rise and that the overall unemployment rate will remain broadly constant. They argue that 'while the unskilled labour pool is smaller, slower growth means that the demand for labour is correspondingly lower. These two effects offset one another leaving the unemployment rate essentially unchanged' (ibid. 879).

What can be learned from these macroeconomic modelling exercises?

So where does this leave our understanding of the macroeconomic impact of AIDS? In a rather confused state, to say the least. The ING-Barings and BER models come to similar conclusions about the likely impact on growth, unemployment and rising per capita income – but they do so via different economic channels. The Arndt and Lewis model not only highlights a different set of economic dynamics, but concludes that the impact on growth will be bigger, and that the final impact of AIDS on per capita income will be negative.

Part of the confusion arises from the workings of the different theoretical underpinnings of the macroeconomic models. Macroeconomic modelling entails imposing a theoretical framework on a set of economic data, and then using the model to project forward in time (or to simulate the impact of economic shocks). The key point is that very different theoretical models assuming different relations between economic variables can all generate a good 'fit' with the current (and historical) data, but produce very different predictions and results from simulations.

In the case of the three macroeconomic models discussed here, a key difference is the way in which they model the economic impact of higher government expenditure. As discussed above, the Arndt and Lewis model assumes that government borrowing crowds out private investment and lowers growth over the longer term. In the more Keynesian models of ING-Barings and BER, the increase in government spending is assumed to support growth by keeping consumption buoyant. ING-Barings in fact argues that if the government maintains strict fiscal discipline in the face of the AIDS pandemic (i.e. does not allow the deficit to rise as a proportion of the GDP) then this would serve to drain demand even faster out of the economy, thus dragging down GDP (and government revenues) in a 'downward spiral' (2000: 22). The Arndt and Lewis model, by contrast, assumes that such a downward spiral would not happen because private investment would increase.

Such differences have major implications for government policy. One theoretical approach implies that borrowing in order to finance increased health expenditure supports growth, the other implies the reverse. And in the absence of any clear way of evaluating the different models, policy makers are left in a state of befuddlement over how to respond at the fiscal level.

But differences between the models also arise as a result of the lack of adequate information about key behavioural coefficients in the models: how much will total factor productivity fall and to what extent will the available pool of labour become less effective? According to the model by Bell *et al.* (2003), the long-term impact of AIDS will be catastrophic because AIDS undermines the incentive and capacity of households to invest in education as well as the transmission of skills across the generations. The model's apocalyptic vision is unconvincing (and its empirical demographic and economic base is weak), but the point about the long-term impact on growth of falling labour productivity is a good one. The size and distribution of this effect, however, remains an open question. Other questions include how will households realign their spending priorities in the face of AIDS? How much more expensive will labour become for firms? To what extent will they be able to pass on the higher costs in the form of price increases? And will investment rise in response to incentives to become more capital-intensive, or will investors take their money out of the country? Any macroeconomic modelling exercise has to make judgements about all of these choices – and in each case the estimate could be wildly off track. As Over (1992) showed ten years ago, modelling the macroeconomic impact of AIDS in Southern Africa is highly sensitive to assumptions about the prevalence of HIV across skill bands and the proportion of health expenditure that is financed out of savings. This remains true today. One must thus be very cautious about all macroeconomic models of the impact of AIDS. At best, they help us think through the dynamic economic impact of AIDS. At worst, they are a misleading and shaky house of cards.

6.3 The impact of AIDS on firms

One of the weaknesses of the macroeconomic modelling work discussed above is that it operates with a very limited understanding of the way that firms are likely to respond to AIDS. International research on the impact of AIDS on firms tends to draw a distinction between direct and indirect costs.[14] Direct (or 'out-of-pocket') costs include pension and provident fund contributions, service bonuses, absenteeism and sick leave, death and funeral benefits, in-firm medical services, and the costs of recruiting and training replacement workers. Such direct costs for African firms are typically low (Avetin and Huard 2000; McPherson *et al.* 2000; Barnett and Whiteside 2002). Part of the reason for this is the general lack of provision of pension and medical benefits to all workers. In South Africa this is reinforced by the fact that HIV-positive workers appear to be concentrated in the lower skill bands,[15] which do not enjoy the same level of benefit provision as skilled and managerial employees. The total impact on firms will vary depending on factors such as whether firms provide in-house medical facilities, the way in which employment benefits are structured, and the distribution of HIV-positive people across the skill-structure.[16] Research in Kenya indicates that the cost of AIDS as a percentage of profits varied from 0.1% in the case of heavy industry, to 7% in the case of wood processing and transportation (Forsythe and Roberts 1994: 29).

Sometimes it is possible to quantify the indirect impact of AIDS on productivity – i.e. when the output of individual workers can be measured directly. Thus, for example, it was possible to measure the impact of AIDS on tea pickers in Kenya. According to a 2003 study, HIV-positive workers plucked significantly less tea (3.9 kg per day) in the 18 months preceding death (Fox *et al.* 2003). However, in most cases, it is difficult to measure the impact of AIDS on productivity – particularly in cases where illness on the part of an individual worker has a negative impact on other members in the work team and on the work process in general. Such effects are harder (if not impossible) to measure, but are potentially of great importance (Avetin and Huard 2000; Barnett and Whiteside 2002; Stevens 2001). For example, Kennedy in her study of the impact of AIDS on a South African coal mine found that the impact was more discernible 'at the coal face' than it was in the eyes of senior management (2002).

Until recently there were no reliable studies of the impact of AIDS on firms in South Africa. Press reports varied wildly and there was little clear understanding of how different estimates of productivity losses were arrived at (Michael 2000; ABT Associates 2000: 40–1). Fortunately, research into the impact of AIDS on a sugar mill in KwaZulu-Natal (Morris *et al.* 2000; Morris and Cheevers 2000), and synthetic modelling work by Rosen *et al.* (2000), are improving our understanding about the nature of the impact on firms in South Africa.[17] However, this kind of empirical work remains (inevitably) subjective – in terms of both estimating indirect costs and how direct costs are framed and quantified – and difficult to generalise across the entire economy. Booysen and Molelekoa (2001) go some of the way towards rectifying this problem in their survey of firms in the Bloemfontein and Welkom areas. But while this study has the advantage of pooling the results from twenty firms, the results cannot be generalised to the region (only 10% of surveyed firms responded, and most were small to medium-size businesses) let alone to the whole of South Africa.

The standard demographic assumption in South Africa appears to be that individuals who contract HIV live for an additional seven to ten years and that most of the debilitating illness and symptoms are manifest in the last two years of life. The KwaZulu-Natal sugar mill study found that in the two years prior to the men taking retirement (on grounds of ill-health), an average of 27.7 days were lost in each year (Morris *et al.* 2000: 940). Of these, 11.7 days were accounted for by sick leave, 5.4 days by hospitalisation, and 10.6 by visits to the clinic (assuming that each visit to the clinic during work hours resulted in half a day lost).

Taking into account estimates for lost wages (owing to lost days), the costs of hiring and training replacement workers (roughly doubled to proxy for lost productivity resulting from disruption), and limited clinic and hospital-related costs, they estimated the cost of each HIV infection to be roughly three times the annual salary in each of the final two years of employment. No adjustment was made for increased pension or medical aid costs, on the grounds that most (94%) of the HIV-positive workers were in the lowest skill bands (Morris *et al.* 2000: 939). These unskilled workers presumably did not have access to firm-based pension plans, and would have made use of government clinics rather than private medical facilities.[18]

In their modelling work on the impact of AIDS on South African firms, Rosen *et al.* (2000) assume that direct firm-based medical expenditure is low. Instead, they focus on pension benefits, service gratuities and death benefits for HIV-positive workers, costs relating to sick leave, and recruitment and training[19] of replacement workers. These (present value of future) costs come to just under twice the annual salary of workers (see Table 6.3).

Rosen *et al.* (ibid.) use the model to show how medical interventions that increase life expectancy save firms money (by pushing costs further into the future – thus causing them to be discounted more heavily). Their model shows that 'the present value of a new HIV infection would fall by 9% if employees' average life expectancy could be extended by one year, by 25% for a three-year extension, and by 38% if five more years of productive life could be achieved' (ibid. 303). (These results simply reflect the fact that they are applying a 10% discount rate.) The implication is that any treatment costing less than R4,412 that extends productive life by a year would be feasible for those on salaries of R25,000 or lower. For higher-paid (skilled) workers, the upper limit of economically feasible treatment rises to R8,433 and R16,475.

Booysen and Molelekoa (2001) adopt a similar methodology to estimate the impact of AIDS on the twenty firms they surveyed in Bloemfontein and Welkom. Their figures were similar to those reported in Rosen *et al.* (2000). Booysen and Molelekoa estimated that the present value of the cost per AIDS death was R44,319 for unskilled employees, R70,437 for skilled employees, and R190,877 for highly skilled employees (2001: 15). However, the ratio of total costs to annual salary was more sensitive to skills level in the Booysen and Molelekoa study (1.35 for unskilled, 1.27 for skilled, and 2.5 for highly skilled). This appears to be because the information obtained from the survey allowed them to differentiate more clearly than Rosen *et al.* between the different benefits provided for different skill levels. They found that only a quarter of firms offered medical benefits – and in those cases, mostly to skilled workers (2000: 9). Booysen and Molelekoa conclude that the average savings to firms of extending productive life by one year is R5,491 per worker (2001: 16).

Table 6.3 *Rosen* et al.'s *present value of the future costs of a new HIV infection, assuming a seven-year interval between infection and death*

Cost component (2000)	Salary = R25,000	Salary = R50,000	Salary = R100,000
Paid sick leave	R5,741	R11,481	R22,961
Pension benefits	R38,487	R76,974	R15,947
Recruitment/training	R4,313	R4,313	R4,313
Total	R48,540	R92,767	R181,222
Ratio of total costs to annual salary	1.94	1.86	1.81
Savings (life extended by one year)*	R4,412 (9%)	R8,433 (9%)	R16,475 (9%)
Savings (life extended by three years)*	R12,071 (12%)	R23,070 (12%)	R45,067 (12%)
Savings (life extended by five years)*	R18,400 (38%)	R35,166 (38%)	R68,697 (38%)

Source: Rosen *et al.* (2000). * Savings are reductions in the present value of future costs of a new HIV infection due to interventions that extend life by one, three or five years. A discount rate of 10% is used. The figures in parentheses are total savings as a percentage of base-line costs.

Note that the estimates discussed so far take only direct costs into account. Once indirect costs and benefits are factored into the calculation, then the case for life-saving interventions becomes even more compelling for firms. As Rosen *et al.* explain:

The financial benefits of pushing further into the future the types of costs analysed above are only a subset of the overall gains to a company of investing in keeping its workforce as healthy as possible for as long as possible. By retaining skilled and experienced employees for an additional year or years, the company also:

- buys time for drug prices to fall and for medical and social science researchers to develop new ways to treat HIV/AIDS;
- reduces the time managers must spend coping with employee deaths and high turnover;

- reduces the impact on the morale, motivation and concentration of the rest of its workforce of having colleagues fall sick and die; and
- creates more time to implement strategies to cope with the pandemic, such as training replacement employees, shifting to less labour-intensive technologies, and managing the loss of overall workforce skill, experience, institutional memory and cohesion that HIV/AIDS is causing (2000: 303).

When Rosen *et al.* did their study, the cost of HAART for a worker (i.e. over R36,000 a year) was between two and nine times higher than the (direct) benefits to business of providing such medication. However, by mid-2001 the cost of HAART had fallen so much that Medicare (a medical aid company in South Africa) was able to provide HAART and CD4 counts and blood tests for about R800 a month – i.e. about R9,600 a year (Regensberg 2001). If we assume the company absorbs half these costs, then this will amount to R4,800 a year. Assuming a discount rate of 10%, the present value of projected expenditure on antiretrovirals over three years is R13,131 and over five years it is R20,016. As indicated by the data in Table 6.4, this suggests that it is cost-effective for firms to provide access to HAART for their more highly skilled personnel and that the cost (to the company) is only marginally higher than the benefits of extending the lives of less skilled workers for a year According to research by Stevens, there is evidence of companies looking to support HIV-positive employees, 'depending on how valuable the employee is to the company' (2001: 12). However, as discussed above, these results consider only the direct costs of AIDS. Once indirect costs are included, the cost-effectiveness of providing HAART to workers becomes much more compelling. Whether firms appreciate this point, and act accordingly, is of course a different question.

If, following the KwaZulu-Natal sugar mill study, we assume that the indirect cost of AIDS (i.e. on productivity, team-cohesion, etc.) amounts to about 50% of total (direct and indirect) economic costs, then we can double the Rosen *et al.* estimates to include these factors.[20] This will push the Rosen *et al.* estimate for the lowest-paid workers up to R97,080 and make it feasible to provide antiretrovirals even to the low-skilled workers. As can be seen from the figures in parentheses in Table 6.4, doubling the economic costs (as a rough proxy for including indirect costs) renders it economically feasible for firms to treat all workers with antiretrovirals in order to prolong life and minimise disruption.

This kind of exercise illustrates the important point not yet taken into account by macroeconomic modellers – i.e. that firms can react to minimise the impact of AIDS on their businesses. As argued above, firms may choose to provide antiretrovirals to their skilled workers – and perhaps even to all workers – thereby extending the life of the workforce and minimising the disruptive impact on the labour market and patterns of consumption. All three macroeconomic models discussed above assumed that providing HAART was out of the question. While this is understandable with regard to the ING-Barings and Arndt and Lewis studies (because the cost of anti-retrovirals was still high in 2000), it is less understandable with respect to the BER study (as the costs of antiretrovirals had fallen dramatically before the study was published). If firms do react by providing antiretrovirals (as has been the case with Anglo American, Daimler-Benz, Mondi and other large companies since 2002), then all three macroeconomic models will have overestimated the impact of AIDS on the workforce, skills shortages, wages, consumption and medical costs. They would, in other words, have overestimated the impact of AIDS on growth and per capita incomes.

Table 6.4 *Net savings to firms as a result of providing HAART to workers (own calculations)*

	Additional 1 year	Additional 3 years	Additional 5 years
Discounted cost to firms of antiretroviral treatment	R4,800	R13,131	R20,016
Net savings (for salaries of R25,000)	R4,412–R4,800 = –R388 (R4,024)	R12,071–R13,131 = –R1,060 (R11,011)	R18,400–R20,016 = –R1,616 (R16,784)
Net savings (for salaries of R50,000)	R8,433–R4,800 = R3,633 (R12,066)	R23,070–R13,131 = R9,939 (R33,009)	R35,166–R20,016 = R15,150 (R50,316)
Net savings (for salaries of R100,000)	R16,475–R4,800 = R11,675 (R28,150)	R45,067–R13,131 = R31,936 (R77,003)	R68,697–R20,016 = R48,681 (R117,378)

Sources: Calculated from data in Rosen *et al.* (2000), see Table 6.3, and Regensberg (2001), assuming a discount rate of 10%. The figures in parentheses include an estimate for productivity losses (i.e. indirect costs) which doubles the savings shown in Table 6.3.

Another way for firms to respond to the AIDS pandemic is to reduce their exposure to the risks and costs associated with AIDS. According to Rosen and Simon (2002), there is an emerging body of evidence that firms in sub-Saharan Africa are avoiding some of the burdens of AIDS through reducing employee benefits, restructuring employment contracts, outsourcing less skilled jobs, selective retrenchments, and changes in production technologies. All of these changes have implications for the rate and pattern of economic growth. While some of the changes help lower the cost of AIDS to individual firms (by shifting the burden of AIDS from firms to the public sector, workers' families and society at large), the private sector as a whole will still feel the effects – albeit via different routes. As McPherson *et al.* point out, 'as the HIV/AIDS epidemic intensifies, the macroeconomic effects of these rising costs will feed back to affect the employers' output, sales, taxes, or access to social services' (2000: 8). In other words, some direct costs can be passed on to others, but the overall macroeconomic impact cannot be avoided.

In addition to reacting to the risks associated with HIV infection in their workforce, firms will also react to AIDS-related changes in the demand for their products. In a recent publication by J. P. Morgan (2001) entitled *How to AIDS-Proof Your Consumer Portfolio*, investors are advised to avoid companies whose consumers are relatively young and relatively poor – or whose products are luxury goods with a high income-elasticity of demand (because these companies could suffer as expenditure is reallocated towards health spending), or who rely on consumer purchases on credit (as defaults are likely to become more common). This kind of market advice is likely to depress stock prices for such firms and industries – thus sending a signal to entrepreneurs to diversify and gradually shift out of such markets. The JD group (which sells furniture and household appliances) has already concluded that its target South African market is likely to be adversely affected by AIDS, and as a consequence has opened stores in the Czech Republic and Poland in order to protect its rate of return to shareholders (Whiteside and Sunter 2000: 106–7).

In short, the structure of the economy is likely to alter as patterns of demand and profitability shift over time. Such change has not been adequately addressed by the major macroeconomic models, which have instead concentrated on the impact of AIDS on the size of the economy, rather than its structure (De Waal 2003: 9). The models have also not dealt adequately with the impact of AIDS on inequality.

According to De Waal, AIDS is likely to increase inequality in Africa because some commercial farmers will be able to buy up land cheaply from families stricken by AIDS, and employ unskilled labour at low wages

(2003: 11). As discussed in the following section, such developments are unlikely to have an impact on inequality in South Africa. Bell *et al.* (2003) also argue that AIDS is likely to increase inequality. They hypothesise that AIDS orphans will have fewer skills (because the early death of their parents will prevent the transmission of knowledge and productive capacity across the generations) and that fewer household resources will be expended on their education. In the Bell *et al.* model, the impact of AIDS on economic growth and inequality in South Africa will worsen over time. However, as this result derives primarily from theoretical assumptions, it is more an illustration of a possible outcome than a credible prediction of actual outcomes. Section 6.4 explores the possible relationship between AIDS and income distribution in South Africa.

6.4 AIDS and inequality in South Africa

Unlike the rest of Africa, employment in peasant or subsistence agriculture is low in South Africa (Seekings 2000). This is primarily the result of the process of de-agrarianisation under apartheid (see also Chapter 7), but it is also a consequence of South Africa's unfavourable climate for small-scale intensive agriculture. As can be seen in Table 6.5, only 7% of employment in South Africa was in subsistence and small-scale agriculture. Given that such a small proportion of household income is generated by subsistence agriculture, the bulk of this 'employment' is in fact large-scale underemployment.

Most income in South Africa is generated in the labour market, and access to employment is a key determinant of poverty and inequality (Leibbrandt *et al.* 2000). Access to jobs, rather than access to land, is the main driver of inequality. The impact of AIDS on inequality is mediated in large part by how the government and private firms react to the AIDS pandemic by changing the level and type of employment, and the benefits available.

As firms react by decreasing their reliance on unskilled labour (a trend that started before the AIDS pandemic) and by moving out of economic sectors whose customer base comprised lower-income consumers, poor households find themselves doubly disadvantaged. Not only is their access to the labour market becoming ever more tenuous, but the products they purchase are becoming scarcer. Conversely, relatively skilled workers benefit from greater employment opportunities (as production becomes more skill- and capital-intensive) and higher wages (as the relative demand for skilled labour increases). They are also living longer and more productive lives as firms provide them with access to antiretroviral treatment. The size of the pie may have shrunk as a result of AIDS, but the employed (especially skilled) workers are enjoying a growing share.

Table 6.5 *South Africa's structure of employment (February 2002 Labour Force Survey)*

	Estimate	%
Non-agricultural formal sector	7,036,000	62%
Commercial agriculture	734,000	6%
Subsistence or small-scale agriculture	792,000	7%
Informal sector	1,767,000	16%
Domestic service	972,000	9%
Total employed	11,393,000	100%

Source: Statistics South Africa, PO210 September 2002

South Africa is increasingly divided along class lines with the gap between the employed and unemployed being of major importance (Seekings and Nattrass 2004). The horrifying element that AIDS brought to the picture is that the divide has also meant the difference between life and death for many people. Those without access to jobs (especially good jobs) have borne the brunt of the AIDS pandemic and will continue to do so until a national treatment plan has been fully rolled out.

Table 6.6 *South Africans' perceptions of primary divisions in the country*

	White	Coloured	Indian	African	Total
Between political parties	21.3%	18.1%	17.4%	22.8%	22.1%
Between rich and poor	29.7%	37.1%	34.0%	29.1%	30.0%
Between people living with HIV/AIDS and the rest	8.9%	9.7%	8.6%	16.1%	14.4%
Between different religions	5.5%	7.5%	6.2%	7.2%	7.0%
Between races	29.3%	21.9%	24.3%	18.2%	20.2%
Between languages	5.3%	5.0%	9.5%	6.6%	6.3%
	100.0%	100.0%	100.0%	100.0%	100.0%

Source: Reconciliation Barometer, Institute for Justice and Reconciliation

According to the 2003 *Reconciliation Barometer* survey, more South Africans believe that the gap between rich and poor is the primary division in society than believe that race is the key division (see Table 6.6). This is to be expected, given the declining importance of racial differences in driving inequality in South Africa (Seekings and Nattrass 2004). It is also worth noting, however, that almost as many Africans highlighted the division between people living with HIV/AIDS and those not infected with the virus, as highlighted racial differences. The AIDS pandemic seems to be affecting perceptions of social solidarity in ways that have yet to be appreciated by researchers or policy makers.

The economic impact of providing HAART

Chapter 4 argued that the public provision of HAART would cost a great deal in terms of direct costs, but that this would partially be compensated for by reduced demands on the health sector because of the lower associated expenditure on AIDS-related opportunistic infections. There are, however, broader macroeconomic benefits to be had from providing HAART. As noted above, HIV-positive workers on HAART are able to lead longer, more productive lives, thus reducing training and other productivity-related costs to the private sector. The same, of course, applies to efficiency within the public sector. According to all three macroeconomic models discussed above, reducing these productivity-related costs will boost economic growth – and thus also tax revenues accruing to the government.

The other potential macroeconomic benefit of HAART relates to consumption. However, as is clear from the discussion of the macroeconomic models, the impact of AIDS on consumption depends on the theoretical underpinnings of the model and the assumptions made about the composition of demand. Demand will fall in some sectors of the economy (e.g. in those market segments catering for durable consumption demand by poorer people), but rise in other sectors (e.g. health care, and in those sectors catering for skilled workers, whose wages will probably rise as the economy restructures). The overall impact on total expenditure (i.e. aggregate demand) is also dependent on whether private sector investment is undermined (e.g. as a result of lower demand and/or increased public-sector borrowing) or boosted (by firms trying to become more capital-intensive and less dependent on unskilled labour). Increases in taxation (to pay for the treatment programme) will reduce disposable income, thus further impacting on the level of demand. If resources are instead drawn away from other government expenditure categories (e.g. defence or education) then the knock-on effect of this on overall consumption demand must also be taken into account. Given that the impact of AIDS on the overall level of consumption is unclear, it follows that the macroeconomic benefits of a national HAART programme are similarly unclear.

Furthermore, we have no way of knowing whether the broader economic benefits of HAART (in terms of averting the AIDS-related shifts in consumption and averting the negative impact of AIDS on productivity) will offset the costs (of higher government expenditure on health and thus higher levels of taxation). The models that assume that higher government expenditure will 'crowd-out' private investment will predict lower net economic benefits than the models that do not make this assumption.

Figure 6.1 traces some of the macroeconomic pathways that may be affected by a public programme to provide HAART. Note that it only

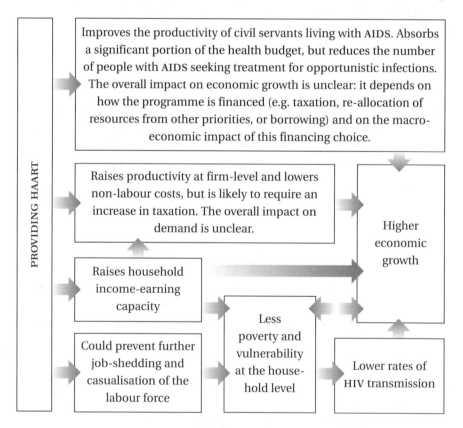

Figure 6.1 *The broader macroeconomic benefits of providing HAART for people living with AIDS*

examines the impact on economic growth – not per capita economic growth. As discussed earlier, the macroeconomic models come to different conclusions about whether the slow-down in economic growth resulting from AIDS will be greater or smaller than that for the population. For models that predict per capita incomes will rise because of AIDS, an implication is that extending the lives of people with AIDS may result in lower overall per capita incomes. The greater the proportion of unemployed people among those receiving HAART, the more likely is this scenario.

An important question concerns the division of responsibility between the private and public sectors for the provision of HAART. Until late 2003 the only means of accessing HAART was through pilot programmes (such as that run by MSF in Khayelitsha) and the private sector. According to one estimate, in 2003 only 20,000 people were accessing HAART in the private sector (AIDS Law Project and TAC 2003). This is a tiny fraction of the over 600,000 AIDS cases projected that year by the ASSA2000 Interventions Model.

As argued earlier, the HAART burden borne by the private sector may well (at least in part) pay for itself in terms of higher productivity, etc. Nevertheless, the private provision of HAART represents an additional non-wage labour cost and as such acts as a disincentive to employ labour. Given the close correlation between unemployment and poverty, such job shedding is socially undesirable. There may thus be a case for the full 'socialisation' of HAART through the rapid expansion of a public-sector treatment programme.

The large pharmaceutical companies typically earn super-profits from the sale of antiretrovirals to the private sector. According to an expert affidavit in support of a 2003 complaint to South Africa's Competition Commission, antiretroviral prices charged to the private sector are between two and four times the estimated cost of research and development plus licensing fees, manufacturing costs and a 16% profit margin (AIDS Law Project and TAC 2003: 41–2). Given that the pharmaceutical companies have proved willing to reduce their prices substantially when supplying government health services – particularly when bargaining is accompanied by the threat of compulsory licensing (Luccini *et al.* 2003) – there is scope for significant reductions in the per patient price of HAART.

In October 2003, former US President Bill Clinton brokered a deal with four generic drug companies (three Indian and one South African) to produce Trizivir, a single-pill triple-drug combination. This could reduce the price of HAART by two thirds (to R81 per patient per month). But to achieve this, voluntary licences have to be negotiated with the patent holders or the government has to issue a compulsory licence.

If the cost of treatment was socialised through a universal publicly funded HAART programme, employers and workers would pay higher taxes but their medical aid premiums would be lower. Whether they would be net beneficiaries of the change depends on the extent of the price differential between the public and private provision of antiretrovirals, and on the extent to which the treatment programme is financed out of an increase in tax (rather than expenditure cuts in other areas), and on the extent to which providing HAART is beneficial for economic growth. However, given that less than 20% of the population was covered by medical aid schemes in 2003, it is likely that employed workers would pay more in taxation if a publicly funded universal HAART programme was introduced than they would in medical aid contributions if one was not. However, the fact that a universal public HAART programme has some benefits for them (i.e. lower medical aid contributions) means that this potential conflict of interest between the employed and the unemployed over AIDS treatment policy could be meliorated to some extent. Although employed workers will probably be net contributors, the burden may not be large enough to encourage them to turn their back on the suffering of others less fortunate than themselves. The preferences of workers on this issue can only be known through a process of social deliberation on how society should respond to the AIDS pandemic.

On sacrificing generations

Whether the impact of AIDS on the economy is to reduce or increase per capita income may have important implications for policy. One could (just about) imagine the relevant authorities examining a macroeconomic model that predicts rising per capita incomes and concluding that AIDS is 'welfare-enhancing' because the size of the economic pie is shrinking slower than the population, thus resulting in a greater piece of the pie for the survivors. Taking this (nasty) thought experiment further, one could imagine someone observing wryly that the AIDS pandemic will help solve the unemployment and poverty problem (because the bulk of AIDS sufferers are poor and unemployed) and thus arguing in favour of a very limited, tokenistic, HAART programme. Rather than extend the lives of as many people living with AIDS as possible, the logic of this particular thought experiment is to kill them off as fast as possible given the constraints of political expediency and the need to at least appear to be concerned about human rights.

There are various ways of responding to such a position. One could dispute the (implicit or explicit) macroeconomic model which underpins it, and point to alternative models predicting that AIDS will result in a fall in per capita incomes. Alternatively, one could argue that the appropriate framework for making a decision is to compare the impact on economic growth of letting the AIDS pandemic take its course with the impact on growth of treating all people living with AIDS. That means engaging in an explicit economic modelling of the paths outlined in Figure 6.1. Unfortunately this is an even more difficult modelling job. The strongest (and I would argue, the most appropriate) response is to challenge the moral basis of any calculation which concludes explicitly or implicitly that one group of people (in this case, the bulk of the generation of HIV-positive people) should be 'sacrificed' for the good of the rest. What kind of argument, one could ask, is that? What does it do for our humanity and concept of society? Should we even be thinking along these lines?

In 1729 Jonathan Swift (author of *Gulliver's Travels* and Dean of St Patrick's Cathedral in Dublin) attempted to shock the English and Irish elite out of their complacency about Irish poverty. So he wrote a satire entitled *A Modest Proposal* in which he argued that children should be sold on the market for food – thus overcoming the problem of poverty and over-rapid population growth in one go. Here is a quote from his argument:

I have already computed the charge of nursing a beggar's child (in which list I reckon all cottagers, labourers, and four fifths of the farmers) to be about two shillings per annum, rags included; and I believe no gentleman would repine to give ten shillings for the carcass of a good fat child. Those who are more thrifty (as I must confess the times require) may flay the carcass; the skin of which artificially dressed will make admirable gloves for ladies, and summer boots for fine gentlemen ... And the money will circulate among ourselves, the goods being entirely of our own growth and manufacture (Swift 1729: 2–4).

Swift's objective was to show in stark form that a humanitarian response to the Irish crisis was necessary. It was a direct challenge to politicians:

After all, I am not so violently bent upon my own opinion as to reject any offer proposed by wise men, which shall be found equally innocent, cheap and effectual. But before something of that kind shall be advanced in contradiction to my scheme, and offering a better, I desire the author or authors will be pleased maturely to consider two points. First, as things now stand, how they will be able to find food and raiment for a hundred thousand useless mouths and backs. And secondly, there being a round million of creatures in human figure throughout this kingdom, whose whole subsistence put into a common stock would leave them in debt two millions of pounds sterling, adding those who are beggars by profession to the bulk of farmers, cottagers and labourers, with their wives and children who are beggars in effect: I desire those politicians who dislike my overture and may perhaps be so bold as to attempt an answer, that they will first ask the parents of these mortals, whether they would not at this day think it a great happiness to have been sold for food, at a year old in the manner I prescribe, and thereby have avoided such a perpetual scene of misfortunes as they have since gone through by the oppression of landlords, the impossibility of paying rent without money or trade, the want of common sustenance, with neither house nor clothes to cover them from the inclemencies of the weather, and the most inevitable prospect of entailing the like or greater miseries upon their breed forever (1729: 4).

Is not such a moral challenge necessary today with regard to the AIDS crisis? Stephen Lewis (the UN secretary general's special envoy for HIV/AIDS in Africa) argued that the seeming lack of political will on the part of the international community to help with the AIDS crisis in the developing world was 'mass murder by complacency' (*Sunday Independent*, 12 January 2003). In his various passionate appeals for action, he constantly stressed the moral imperative to act in order to alleviate human suffering. Justice Edwin Cameron, South Africa's highest profile HIV-positive activist, similarly placed the value of human life and dignity at the centre of his argument in favour of providing HAART:

[T]he calculus of disease and death from AIDS renders all the evasive counter-rhetoric dramatically unconvincing. None of it is persuasive when the brute fact is brought home that life is available and within reach, but is being denied to those who crave it (2001: 6–7).

His challenge to society is to grasp the nettle of the value of a human life and put that into the calculation as well. Rather than look at the health costs alone, society should be asking why money is being spent on armaments and a presidential jet rather than on HAART. It is to the credit of civil society organisations (like TAC) that these questions have been posed in the public arena.

Once questions are posed in this way, the focus falls on the entire ambit of government policies. How government policy affects the generation of income and wealth – and thus the resources available for redistribution by means of taxation and government spending – becomes pertinent to addressing AIDS. How private sector investors are likely to respond to AIDS policy also needs to be considered. Would they have been put off by the increase in the budget deficit and/or taxation, or would they have been impressed by the dedicated and professional response to a national health emergency? Would businesses have been annoyed by increased taxation, or would they have been relieved by the fact that less of their workers were taking sick leave and subsequently dying? Would national savings have been lowered by the increased demands of government borrowing and taxation, or would national savings have been raised because less money would have been spent by people on funerals and on rushing sick children and adults to hospitals and clinics?

The government's restrictive fiscal policy framework (GEAR),[21] which has structured South Africa's growth strategy since 1996, assumes that reducing taxation, spending and the deficit is required to boost savings and investment (Nattrass 1996). This has resulted in a falling budget deficit, but has also probably contributed to slower growth than would have been the case if a less restrictive stance had been adopted (Weeks 1999). Although the 2003/2004 budget was mildly expansionary and contained extra resources for combating AIDS, South Africa's use of the budget as an instrument to address AIDS remains cautious. Given the finance minister's statements in favour of spending additional resources on growth-enhancing items (such as education) rather than HAART,[22] it would appear that his basic position on AIDS treatment is that it is an unproductive form of consumption expenditure which if rolled out on a large scale would threaten the underpinnings of his growth strategy. He appears not to see combating AIDS as a form of social investment, or as a reasonable priority which, if necessary, requires an increase in taxation. He probably assumes that income earners (workers and employers) would prefer lower taxation and less expenditure on AIDS, to higher taxation and a more universal approach to providing HAART. Chapter 7 argues that AIDS is too impor-tant a social issue for such an assumption to be left in the hands of the finance minister. It should be the product of broad social deliberation about how society should respond to the moral challenges posed by AIDS.

7 Conclusion

In the late 1990s, when AIDS activists and medical practitioners first started demanding a national MTCTP programme, the government said it was 'unaffordable'. This discourse remained hegemonic even after studies were published (and presented in the form of affidavits) showing that the health sector would almost certainly *save* money by implementing such a programme. It was only after being ordered to do so by the Constitutional Court in 2002, that the government started rolling out MTCTP. The discourse of unaffordability was also used to justify the government's initial refusal to provide HAART through the public sector. But as it became clear during the course of 2003 that public pressure and political expediency were making this inevitable, government discourse shifted in subtle ways. Rather than arguing that HAART was simply unaffordable, the government highlighted the complexities of AIDS treatment, and the need for effective and 'sustainable' interventions. A sustainable programme, which by definition grows in line with available resources, is obviously desirable. The key question which is being begged through the use of this term, however, is the level of resource commitment from the government.

HAART is very expensive, and although there are significant savings to the health budget (relating to lower AIDS-related morbidity and mortality), these are unlikely to outweigh the direct costs of a national HAART intervention. As shown in Chapter 4, expanding an AIDS intervention to include the provision of HAART for all those who need it will have substantial benefits in terms of fewer orphans, fewer new HIV infections and longer life-expectancy. However, it will require the mobilisation of significant resources. These will either have to be raised through taxation, or reallocated away from other spending priorities. There are, in other words, serious issues of social choice involved.

7.1 The moral challenge posed by AIDS for society

South Africa can 'afford' a large-scale AIDS intervention (which includes HAART) in the sense that it will absorb only a small fraction of national income (between 1% and 3% of GDP according to the calculations presented in Chapter 4). But affordability cannot be determined with reference to cost calculations alone. There are always competing demands on scarce resources and the crucial issue is rather whether society wishes to allocate resources in this manner. Do we want to pay higher taxation and ensure that a set of AIDS interventions is sufficiently well resourced that it reaches all who need it, or would we prefer a limited AIDS treatment intervention, which, by definition, reaches only a few? Do we make the necessary sacrifices to treat everyone, or do we create a situation in which limited resources require the application of triage and rationing?

Richard Rorty (1996) argues that if society lacks the political will to help those in need, then the notion of a moral community of citizens is empty. He discusses this with respect to the American underclass, but the resonance with the South African AIDS issue is clear:

When a hospital is deluged with an impossibly large flood of victims of a catastrophe, the doctors and nurses begin to perform triage: they decide which of the victims are 'medically feasible' – which ones are appropriate recipients of the limited medical resources available. When the American underclass is told that it is politically unfeasible to remedy their situation, they are in the same situation as the accident victims who are told that it is unfeasible to offer them medical treatment.

In both cases, those who make the decision about feasibility are answering the question 'who are we' by excluding certain human beings from membership in 'we, the ones who can hope to survive'. When we realise that it is unfeasible to rescue a person or group, it is as if they had already gone before us into death. Such people are, as we say, 'dead to us'. Life, we say, is for the living.

For the sake of their own sanity, and for the sake of the less grievously wounded patients who *are* admitted to the hospital, the doctors and nurses must simply blank out on all those moaning victims who are left outside in the street. They must cease to think about them, pretend they are already dead. These doctors and nurses illustrate the point that if you cannot render assistance to the people in need, your claim that they form part of your moral community is empty (1996: 4).

This suggests that those who fail to be reached because of a limited (rather than universal) treatment programme are in effect excluded from South Africa's moral community. A similar point was made in 1989 by a Brazilian AIDS activist who argued that failure to provide treatment condemned AIDS sufferers to 'civil death' (cited in Galvao 2002: 1863). Two years later the Brazilian government provided Zidovudine (AZT) through the public health system and, in 1996, the Brazilian president (Fernando Henrique Cardoso) signed a law establishing free distribution of drugs to people living with AIDS. By contrast, it took until late 2003 for the South African government to accept that HAART should be provided in the public sector but, even then, its commitment was highly qualified by concerns relating to resource constraints.

The South African cabinet may believe that, for macroeconomic reasons, taxation should not be increased and that there is insufficient room in the existing budget for reallocating resources to provide universal access to HAART. Alternatively, it may think that there is insufficient public support to fund anything more than a limited treatment roll-out. It is even possible that the government's initial reluctance to accept even the need for antiretrovirals was because of President Mbeki's views on AIDS, and that the cautious approach to a treatment roll-out is an ongoing legacy of this. It is, in short, unclear why the South African government prevaricated for so long on the treatment issue, or why it has subsequently adopted such a cautious and qualified approach to providing it. What is clear, however, is that there has been no serious public discussion about what *scale* of response is appropriate to combat the AIDS pandemic. Instead, the implicit and explicit choices which have been, and continue to be, made on behalf of citizens have been disguised by a rhetoric of technical and economic expertise. AIDS treatment, we are told, has to be rolled out cautiously and slowly because it is 'complex' and we need careful planning to ensure 'sustainability'. This rhetoric portrays the government's slow and limited treatment intervention as purely a technical issue – when in fact it reflects a set of judgements about what scale of intervention is appropriate. Given the important implications for society, there is a compelling case for a much broader and more open discussion of precisely this issue.

How could such a process of social deliberation be brought about? One option is to go down the route of direct democracy by educating the public about the various options and then holding a referendum. An alternative approach would be to build on South Africa's tradition of social corporatism and make better use of the peak-level bargaining institution, NEDLAC. The main beneficiaries of NEDLAC have so far been labour and business, but there is potential (via the 'development chamber') to involve a wider range of civil society groupings in discussions over key policy interventions including AIDS. Ideally this should be accompanied by a public education campaign and the development of local level discussion forums (modelled, perhaps, on the Irish social accord process).

As discussed in Chapter 2, AIDS policy has already been the subject of negotiation in NEDLAC. Between July and December 2002, representatives of government, labour and business negotiated a 'framework agreement' in favour of a treatment plan. The process broke down when the government refused to sign the agreement – saying variously that there was no agreement, or that, as the government, it was not required to sign anything of the sort. This had the unfortunate effect of undermining NEDLAC and forcing TAC to confront the government through legal action and via high profile civil disobedience campaigns in 2003. By undermining, rather than building on the strengths of NEDLAC, the government lost an opportunity to engage in a process of social consensus-building on how South Africa should respond to the AIDS pandemic.

The advantage of an open and transparent bargaining process is that it forces representatives of civil society to lay bare their notions of who is (and who is not) part of the 'moral community'. Although each party brings a set of interests to the table, the bargaining process itself has the potential to transform attitudes and positions. As O'Donnel remarks about the highly participatory and broad-ranging Irish social accord process:

Bargaining describes a process in which each party comes with definite preferences and seeks to maximise their gains. While this is a definite part of Irish social partnership, the overall process (including various policy forums) would seem to involve something more. Partnership involves the players in a process of deliberation that has the potential to shape and reshape their understanding, identity and preferences (2001: 5).

Perhaps this potential for policy forums to shape and reshape preferences is because they encourage 'reasonable' discussion about how to construct a just and fair social order – as suggested by Rawls (see Chapter 1). To quote him once more:

[I]t is by the reasonable that we enter as equals the public world of others and stand ready to propose, or to accept, as the case may be, fair terms of co-operation with them ... Insofar as we are reasonable, we are ready to work out the framework for the public social world (1993: 53).

It is, of course, possible that after reasoned reflection and discussion about universal access to HAART in South Africa, the decision might weigh against providing treatment on a large enough scale to reach all who need it. This would be the case, for example, if most participants believed that AIDS-victims are responsible for their own predicament and that, for this reason, the state has no moral duty to treat them; that the public health benefits are not sufficiently compelling to justify the expense; and that the resources required could better promote social justice if allocated elsewhere. However, reasonable people may decide that the social benefits of

HAART far exceed the sum of the individual benefits to HAART patients, and hence that, irrespective of moral desert, it makes sense to provide treatment to all who need it (and as soon as possible). They may, for that matter, simply decide that there are no valid ethical arguments for effectively excluding anyone with AIDS from the 'moral community' – and hence that universal access to AIDS treatment needs to be guaranteed and funded out of additional taxation. One cannot predict the outcome of a social process of deliberation. The point is simply that such a process is preferable to one in which social choices are made by the government and disguised as technical issues.

As also noted in Chapter 1, the institutional context shapes social values, and self-interested behaviour is ever present. When competing social objectives are constrained by scarce resources, and where different social interests are served by different policies, working out the framework for the public social world will not be a simple process. In South Africa's case, social values and solidarity are likely to be sorely tested by the challenges posed by AIDS.

If the AIDS pandemic is perceived as being likely to result in an increase in per capita income, then the elite may regard it as in their best interests to do very little of significance to halt the pandemic or alleviate its consequences. Those with the economic means to better protect themselves and their families against HIV infection (by providing access to education, condoms, healthy diets and safer lifestyle choices), and who have access to medical schemes to treat themselves and their loved ones if they become infected, may think their interests are better served by a 'do-very-little' scenario. They may privately calculate that they stand to benefit more as individuals from a set of policies that prioritises economic growth and minimises taxation, than they would from a social response that includes rapid universal access to HAART and entails higher taxation and spending cuts in other areas. They would, of course, be wrong to think that they can entirely insulate themselves in this way from the AIDS pandemic. But if they believe they can, this course of action may seem preferable.

This has implications for social solidarity regarding AIDS treatment. For example, organised labour may well baulk at the tax implications of a full-scale tax-financed AIDS intervention. Many workers are already able to access HAART through their employers or medical aids and most live in urban areas (which are at the front of the queue in the treatment roll-out because the greatest capacity to deliver treatment is in the large urban hospitals). Employed workers may thus have an incentive to support a limited roll-out (with correspondingly less onerous tax implications for their pay packets) rather than a large-scale intervention aimed at reaching all those who need it.

The structural problem at the root of this social tension is South Africa's high unemployment rate (see Chapter 4). This is a function of South Africa's skill- and capital-intensive growth path, the decline of the mining industry, and the fact that unlike most other African countries, South Africa lacks a significant peasant agricultural sector. Most employment is in the formal sector, and for the past two decades this sector has not been able to generate enough jobs to prevent unemployment from rising (Nattrass 2003a).

Implicit in the notion of the 'development dilemma' posed by AIDS is the assumption that AIDS is killing off productive adults, i.e. the very human resources needed to grow the economy (see Chapter 1). But what if over a third of the labour force cannot find gainful employment, as has been the case in South Africa for almost a decade? Under such circumstances, the economic elite may believe it can 'afford' to let the AIDS pandemic run its course through poor, high-unemployment areas, while relying primarily on the market to allocate HAART to productive workers. Chapter 6 argued that business has an incentive to supply HAART to its workforce (especially the skilled), while at the same time reducing dependence on unskilled labour. This will alter the nature of the growth path, but it will still generate growth (albeit in the context of high and probably rising unemployment). In such conditions, the government will be under no growth-related pressure to provide government-funded universal access to HAART treatment.

This may have been one of the reasons for the South African government's reluctance to embark on AIDS treatment interventions and its subsequent limited and gradualist approach. It is even hypothetically possible that the government's initial refusal to implement MTCTP – a policy stance that was widely regarded as both immoral and irrational – was informed by a fear that this would be the foot in the door for AIDS treatment. The government may have made a strategic decision to resist all programmes using antiretrovirals in order to stave off the day when pressure from civil society to treat all people living with AIDS could no longer be resisted. If this kind of hard economic calculus is an aspect of government decision making on AIDS, then this is all the more reason to place AIDS policy making in the public domain and to ensure adequate representation of civil society in any bargaining/consultation process about the scale and pace of implementation of HAART.

7.2 Alleviating poverty and addressing AIDS

Let us assume for the moment that a representative consultative forum was in place to discuss the appropriate scale of an AIDS prevention and treatment intervention. The big question which is likely to present itself at the outset is how best to allocate resources between poverty alleviation and combating AIDS. Chapter 4 touched on this issue with regard to the trade-off between disability grants and HAART. It was pointed out that access to HAART may pose real dilemmas for those individuals who are currently accessing the disability grant as a result of AIDS-sickness. One option is to provide a smaller (rather than no) grant for those on HAART, because, although many of them are now physically capable of work, the chances of finding it are slim. But this raises the obvious question of why society is not making provision for *all* unemployed or poor South Africans.

In Chapter 1 it was observed that the demand for a 'right to subsistence' has characterised popular protest across countries and over the course of history. As Scott puts it, 'this right is surely the minimal claim that an individual makes on his society and is perhaps the reason it has such moral force' (1976: 177). Arguments in favour of a universal basic income grant (BIG) for all citizens can be located within this tradition of moral economy. As indicated below, there are strong arguments for supporting a BIG in South Africa. A BIG will absorb a significant share of government resources, but it has many advantages that are of relevance to the development dilemma posed by AIDS. Addressing poverty directly by channelling income into the hands of the poor thus helps lower the spread of HIV. Of course there are many other ways of addressing poverty – most notably through economic policies that boost growth, particularly in labour-intensive sectors (Seekings and Nattrass 2004). However, in order to simplify the discussion and maintain a focus on what can be done directly through the budget, this chapter considers only direct welfare interventions to alleviate poverty.

South Africa's welfare system provides for the young (through child grants), the elderly (through generous non-contributory pensions) and the disabled. The underlying assumption is one of full-employment, i.e. that able-bodied adults can provide for themselves through work (Nattrass and Seekings 1997). In the absence of any welfare support for the unemployed, the burden of supporting the unemployed falls on pensioners and those with jobs.

Welfare support for the unemployed could be provided in two ways: via a means-tested system (a 'dole'); or through a universal BIG. The advantage of the latter is that it wastes fewer resources on bureaucracy. A BIG of R100 per month for all South Africans could contribute substantially to reducing poverty and inequality in South Africa. According to Bhorat (2002), the numbers of people living below the poverty line would fall by about two thirds. Interestingly there appears to be widespread support for the introduction of a BIG in South Africa, ranging from the opposition Democratic Alliance to the socialist left (Matisonn and Seekings 2002). But there is less agreement about how to finance it. The recent 'Taylor Committee' report on comprehensive welfare reform argued in favour of a BIG (Taylor Committee 2002), but was curiously silent about how it should be financed.

The 'People's Budget'[1] (supported by COSATU, the South African Council of Churches and the South African NGO Coalition) proposes that part of the needed revenue could be raised through a 'solidarity levy' in the form of a 17.5% surcharge on income tax for the top two quintiles – and the rest in the form of increased taxation of 'the high income group'. This is broadly in line with the COSATU 7th National Congress resolution that the cost of the BIG must 'fall on the rich'. By contrast, Le Roux (2002) proposes that the BIG be financed by a 7.3 percentage point increase in VAT and a 50% increase in excise and fuel taxes. The advantage of Le Roux's proposal is that it is broad-based and redistributive. Those who spend more than R1,000 a month end up paying more in consumption taxes than they gain from the R100 universal grant.

Despite popular support for a BIG, the South African government has been reluctant to endorse it. One source of concern is the 'hand-out' nature of the grant, which in many circles (including the government) is deemed less desirable than providing people with the 'dignity of work' through direct job creation.[2] Those who believe that citizens have an obligation to work are also opposed to a BIG. Another concern, perhaps, is that the R100 a month grant, once implemented, could become a political site of struggle over the size of the grant. As Le Roux (2002) has shown, the net cost of a BIG (financed out of VAT) will be about R15 billion a year, i.e. a few billion more than the government is currently spending on the gross cost of old age pensions. If the grant were to double or treble (as a result of demands from voters), then the cost implications would be serious indeed.

There are, of course, other ways of channelling income into the hands of the unemployed. An obvious alternative to a grant is to 'self-target' the unemployed by offering low-wage jobs through a government-funded national public works programme (PWP). Low-wage PWPs target the poor (because only the poor will work for low wages) without undermining the labour market. Properly designed PWPs have the potential to alleviate poverty (McCord 2002) and have the additional benefit of creating assets (e.g. building roads, removing alien vegetation from watercourses, etc.). The disadvantage of PWPs (relative to a BIG) is that a substantial pro-portion of resources (typically between 40–50%) are absorbed by administration – rather than being channelled more directly to the poor via wages. The more complex the PWP (e.g. those that attempt to provide some skills training as well), the greater the proportion of resources is absorbed by management, and the greater the risk of inefficiency and failure.

Nevertheless, the experience of Chile has shown that it is possible to absorb a high proportion of the unemployed in government-funded and managed PWPs (Cortaza 1997).[3] According to McCord (2003), it would cost South Africa R22.8 billion to provide low wage employment for 2.6 million unemployed people a year[4] (i.e. about one third of the 7.7 million who report that they do not have jobs and would like one). This is more than the net cost of a BIG (which, as noted above, Le Roux (2002) estimates to be in the region of about R15 billion a year) and about the same as the (mid-point estimate of) the cost of the full-scale AIDS intervention including HAART (Chapter 4).

But whether the South African state has the capacity at all levels of government to implement such a national PWP successfully, however, is a good question. Scandals concerning corruption and inefficiency in the delivery of pensions in the Eastern Cape indicate that in poorer parts of the country such capacity is likely to be lacking. This is a major problem from the point of view of inequality because it is precisely these areas that require well-targeted and well-designed PWPs the most. One of the big limitations of PWPs is the high proportion of expenditure that gets chan-nelled to the bureaucrats administering the projects rather than to the wages of the beneficiaries. If the bureaucrats do not do a good job to ensure that the PWPs reach the poorest people quickly and efficiently, the redistributive impact is seriously weakened. Under the circumstances, then, it is likely that a BIG will be better targeted than a national PWP, and is likely to reach more of the poor, and more effectively. A BIG has the added advantage in the context of the AIDS pandemic of reaching those who are too ill with AIDS to participate in PWPs.

Given that income-earners are beneficiaries of the current growth path, an appropriate social-democratic response may well be higher taxation in order to finance a BIG. Higher taxation was part of the implicit social contract embedded in the Scandinavian social-democratic model. Such 'social accords' sought to balance the need to maintain profitability (so as to encourage investment and ensure sustainable growth) while ensuring a reasonable growth in wage income and the provision of basic income support and training for the unemployed (Nattrass 1999). More recent social accords, e.g. the 'new social accords' forged in Ireland, the Netherlands and Australia during the 1980s and 1990s, focussed on expanding employment and on creating innovative links between labour-market, welfare and economic policies (Rhodes 2001). In each case, organised labour made concessions on labour regulations (so as to expand job creation) in return for skills-development policies and lower taxation. In other words, the focus of the new social accords was on restructuring the economy in order to create more jobs.

If South Africa builds on its tradition of tripartite negotiation and opts for a type of 'new social accord' strategy, then this will have to be without the carrot of lower taxes (Nattrass 2003b). Given the scale of unemployment and the social need for higher welfare and health spending, tax increases for income earners rather than decreases will be the order of the day. The only 'sweetener' which can be offered to organised labour is that by making concessions in order to expand employment, the number of tax payers will increase, thereby sharing the burden more broadly.

In the concluding part of Chapter 4, it was observed that South Africa could finance a full-scale AIDS intervention including HAART by raising VAT[5] by between 3 and 7 percentage points (depending on assumed hospitalisation costs). It is, however, important to remember that the estimated costs of such a large-scale intervention assume a rapid and extensive take-up of HAART. It also includes a substantial estimate of the costs of treating opportunistic infections. If one was, instead, to assume a longer roll-out period, and lower costs of treating opportunistic infections (by assuming that public-sector rationing takes place), then total costs would be lower. Reduced prices for HAART will also lower costs.

According to Le Roux's (2002) estimates, an increase in VAT of 7% is required to finance a BIG.[6] If we assume that both a BIG and a large-scale AIDS intervention (including HAART) were to be implemented, this would (at current antiretroviral prices) require a significant increase in taxation. Assuming the cost estimate reported in Chapter 4, the required tax increase would be in the region of increasing VAT by 10 to 14 percentage points. Is this feasible?

There is no exact technical answer to this question as different societies tolerate different levels of taxation. Welfare expenditure as a proportion of GDP has risen with economic development, and in times of crisis (such as war) citizens have accepted large increases in taxation as legitimate (Seekings 2003a). The notion of what is and is not 'affordable' thus varies according to the social and economic context. Given the scale of the unemployment problem and the AIDS pandemic, it is possible (but probably unlikely) that reasonable South Africans might agree to such an increase in taxation so as to deal with it.

The treasury would of course worry a great deal about the macroeconomic impact of such a tax increase and be unconvinced by any argument to the effect that putting income in the hands of the poor (through a BIG) will counter-balance the negative impact of higher taxation. But the jury is still out on these issues. According to one (albeit rather optimistic) view, South Africa's average tax rate is 'significantly less than that which would be predicted given the country's economic profile' and that 'an additional R25 billion per year could be mobilised without undermining international competitiveness' (Samson 2002b: 91).

Assuming (for the point of argument) that this positive assessment is correct, an additional R25 billion could go a long way towards financing both a BIG and a large-scale AIDS intervention including HAART. Taking Le Roux's (2002) estimate of R15 billion a year for a BIG, and assuming the lower-bound cost estimate of R14.1 billion for the AIDS intervention (see Chapter 4), we would need to find about R4 billion a year in addition to the resources mobilised by the increase in taxation. Following the lead of Botswana, some relief could be sought by applying for grants from the Global Fund for AIDS, TB and Malaria and from other international aid agencies. Cutting South Africa's defence expenditure is another possible source of revenue. However, neither defence cuts nor the Global Fund can be relied on for sustainable funding. Ultimately, South African citizens have to grasp the nettle of higher taxation to fund a large-scale AIDS intervention including treatment for all who need it.

7.3 Why social deliberation is necessary

The central normative thread running through this book is the argument that a broad process of social deliberation is required over AIDS policy and, in particular, over the additional resource requirements needed to fund a large-scale intervention including universal access to HAART. It was argued that the government's rhetoric of expertise was deflecting attention away from the implicit social choices that were being made on behalf of society.

An obvious rejoinder to this is to argue that it is precisely the role of the government to make social choices on behalf of society. Democratic governments which do not allocate resources broadly in line with social preferences, run the risk of being voted out of office. As noted in Chapter 2, one of the reasons why the South African government changed its stance on the provision of HAART in the public sector may well have been concerns about losing ground in the 2004 election if it did not do so. Given that South Africa is a democracy, is it not then appropriate to allow technocrats in the treasury and ministry of health to determine how best to allocate scarce resources? After all, they make resource allocation decisions every day as part of the normal functions of government. What makes AIDS policy different?

AIDS is different because it is a public health crisis, which not only has deep social roots, but challenges the very notion of what it means to be a society. Serious social reflection and debate will not only help raise the consciousness of citizens about AIDS (thereby contributing to prevention), but will help shape a genuine social response to this challenge. AIDS policy is too important to be left in the hands of technocrats.

Notes

1. Introduction

1. Benatar (2002) argues that for practical reasons it is impossible to distinguish between those who are, and who are not, responsible for their condition. His argument was not designed to prevent some categories of people from being treated, but rather to highlight the moral difficulties implicit in the demand for treatment.

2. The most famous academic statement is the Harvard Consensus Statement (2001), signed by members of the Faculty of Harvard University.

3. In July 2002 at the Barcelona International AIDS Conference, the World Health Organisation and other UN organisations committed themselves to the goal of expanding AIDS treatment to three million people in developing countries by 2006, and the Economic Community of West African States has committed itself to providing treatment for 400,000 people by 2005 (Lucchini *et al.* 2003: 173).

4. The Rand is South Africa's currency. In July 2003, $1 could purchase R7.50.

5. Barnett and Whiteside (2002) also provide a useful introduction to the science of AIDS.

6. These estimates are drawn from the ASSA2000 Interventions Model.

7. For a user-friendly introduction to the global AIDS pandemic (its virology, epidemiology and socio-economic impact) see Barnett and Whiteside (2002). Whiteside and Sunter (2000) provide an earlier introduction, focussing specifically on South Africa.

8. Women are between two and four times more likely than men to contract HIV from a sexual encounter. Reasons include higher concentrations of HIV in semen than in vaginal fluid, the larger surface of exposed female genital area, the longer period of exposure of semen in the vaginal tract, and the greater permeability of the mucous membranes in the vagina compared to the penis (see summary of evidence in Baylies and Bujra (2001: 5)).

9. The high rate of HIV prevalence in KwaZulu-Natal has been attributed in part to the trucking routes entering the province from Malawi and Zambia (Williams *et al.* 2000: 129).

10. The practice of dry sex entails the use of cloth and herbs to dry and shrink the vagina. This practice, which is common in Southern Africa, results in abrasions and increased risk of HIV transmission (Wojcicki and Malala 2001: 108–9).

11. This was also found to be the case in a study of migrant men in Carltonville, Johannesburg. Multivariate logistic regression indicated that circumcised men were 30% less likely to be HIV infected (Williams *et al.* 2000: 59, 118).

12. A survey of university students (which included HIV testing) at the Rand Afrikaans University in Johannesburg found HIV prevalence to be 1%, i.e. significantly lower than they expected. The researchers argued that this low level of prevalence can be attributed to high rates of condom use, low levels of sexual activity, high levels

of knowledge about AIDS – all of which are probably a function of the fact that RAU students come from 'relatively well-off families' (Ichharam and Martin 2002: 379). However, as the prevalence test was not random (students were invited to volunteer their 'spit for science'), the lower HIV prevalence could simply reflect selection bias in the sample (if those who were more at risk of HIV infection were more likely to decline the invitation to participate in the survey).

13. Although workers aged over 40 have statistically significantly lower levels of HIV prevalence than younger workers, there is no significant difference between those in their twenties and those in their thirties.

14. Radio report on AM Live, 13 August 2003.

15. See CADRE 2000a: 41–7 for a bibliography of the impact of HIV/AIDS on households. Recent South African survey data indicates that AIDS-affected households draw from savings to finance medical expenditure and funerals (Booysen *et al.* 2001), cut back on food, increase their informal borrowings and rely on relatives (Cross 2001) and cut back on expenditure on clothes, electricity, food and school fees (Steinberg *et al.* 2002a, 2002b). See also Chapter 6.

16. According to a recent South African survey of the impact of AIDS on households, 68% of care-givers were female (Johnson *et al.* 2002).

17. The term is Poku's (Poku 2002).

18. In the 1980s, Cuba tested the entire population for HIV and isolated those found HIV-positive (mainly soldiers returning from the war in Angola) in 'sanitoria'. While this has certainly helped reduce the scale of the AIDS epidemic in Cuba, it raises serious concerns about government control and gross human rights violations (Whiteside and Sunter 2000: 18).

19. In this regard, Rawls follows Sidley's (1953: 560) classic distinction between the reasonable and the rational: 'knowing that people are rational we do not know the ends they will pursue, only that they will pursue them intelligently. Knowing that people are reasonable where others are concerned, we know that they are willing to govern their conduct by a principle from which they and others can reason in common; and reasonable people take into account the consequences of their actions on others' well-being' (Sidley as discussed by Rawls (1993: 49)).

20. Rawls argues that 'rational agents approach being psychopathic when their interests are solely in benefit to themselves' (1993: 51).

2. AIDS policy in South Africa

1. In 1990 the first of a series of random surveys of blood samples of women attending public-sector antenatal clinics found an HIV prevalence rate of 0.8%. By 1991, the figure had doubled to 1.5%, thus providing a clear indication that the AIDS pandemic was beginning to take off.

2. In the 1995/6 financial year, the AIDS Programme spent less than half its allocated funds, and by May 1997 only 13% of European Union funds for AIDS programmes (allocated in 1995) had been spent (Schneider and Stein 2001: 727).

3. For a wide-ranging discussion of the Mbeki presidency, see Jacobs and Calland (2002).

4. The then director general (Ayanda Ntsaluba) made this point at the Durban 2003 AIDS conference and several times on the radio. Nono Simelela, chief director (HIV/AIDS and STDs), has made the point several times at academic conferences, once even bursting into tears when describing how hard it is to work with recalcitrant politicians. In August 2003 she told a workshop at the University of the Witwatersrand that attending academic conferences was frowned upon by her political superiors and that she would not be surprised to find that the National Intelligence Service was keeping tabs on her.

5. See Sparks (2003: 283–95) for a fascinating account of the AIDS dissidents and Mbeki's introduction to their world.

6. Parallel importation occurs if a drug is sold by the patent owner (or licensee) into country A and is then sold on to country B by a third party.

7. Compulsory licensing allows a generic manufacturer to produce a drug before the patent has expired. Usually some royalty is paid to the patent holder.

8. A group of HAART patients on the MSF programme in Khayelitsha responded by writing to Mbeki to explain that the Brazilian drugs were keeping them alive.

9. See Paltiel and Stinnett (1998) for a clear and user-friendly discussion of how economic decision and social choice models can be used to help governments allocate resources towards HIV prevention.

3. Mother-to-child transmission prevention in South Africa

1. Anand and Hanson (1997) argue that this is one of the least attractive features of the DALY and that there are no ethical grounds for the application of such discounting factors. See Murray and Acharya (1997) for a defence of the DALY.

2. This is similar to the results of a study by Kinghorn (1998) showing that cost per DALY is likely to range from $26 to $65.

3. Researchers at Harvard University have compiled various cost-effectiveness studies in the United States to construct 'league tables' as a tool for decision-making. The problem with such tables, however, is that the analyses are not necessarily compatible, and the availability of programmes for inclusion in the table is not random (Paltiel and Stinnett 1998: 140).

4. Economists typically discount costs that occur in the future (to reflect the premium placed on current consumption). Stringer et al. (2000), using information from Marseille et al. (1999), apply a discount factor to medical expenditure

over the life of an HIV-positive child in sub-Saharan Africa and arrive at a figure of $281. This figure is thus less than the cost estimates I adopt here for South Africa for two reasons: (a) costs are lower in poorer countries where treatment is limited, and (b) the costs have been discounted. I have chosen not to adopt a discount rate because it is not clear what discount rate should be used (hence the adoption of a discount rate introduces an arbitrariness to the calculation), and because it makes the final cost figure difficult to grasp at an intuitive level. However, for those who would like to see a discount rate applied, the cost sensitivity analysis – which reduces total hospital costs over the life of an HIV-positive child by 25% – can be regarded as the product of a calculation that discounts future cost by about 4.5% per annum. Given that the results of the sensitivity analysis are still strongly robust, the main conclusion of the analysis presented here is unaffected by the decision not to apply a discount rate to future medical costs.

5. A Durban-based study suggests that exclusive breastfeeding strategies may better protect babies from HIV infection than mixed feeding (breastfeeding and substitute feeding) strategies (Coutsoudis *et al.* 1999; Coutsoudis *et al.* 2001). Some people regard this as conclusive proof that exclusive breastfeeding prevents HIV transmission (e.g. Kuhn 2002a). However, the research design of the Durban study makes it very difficult to draw firm conclusions because it was based on self-reporting from mothers rather than on an experimental design. If as few as four mothers with HIV-positive babies had decided to move to mixed feeding strategies because of the child's failure to thrive, then this source of bias could explain the result (Forsyth 2001). Kuhn (2002b) argues that the researchers tried hard to check for this kind of bias and could not find any proof of it. However, it cannot be ruled out, and for this reason I have argued elsewhere that one should not base policy decisions about exclusive breastfeeding solely on the results of this study (Forsyth and Nattrass 2002).

6. Reported by Costa Gazi at the 'AIDS in Context' conference, University of the Witwatersrand, April 2001.

7. This means that the number of women on the MTCTP programme is reduced by a third. It is assumed further that only two thirds of HIV-positive children ever reach hospitals (hence the 'do nothing' scenario costs less) and that the HIV-positive children born to those women who do not participate in the MTCTP programme never arrive at hospitals either. In other words, only those HIV-positive children of mothers who choose to participate in the MTCTP programme actually get (limited) treatment for opportunistic infections.

8. Information obtained from interviews with physicians at Edendale Hospital, Pietermaritzburg, the Red Cross Children's Hospital, Cape Town, and the Dora Nginza Hospital, Port Elizabeth.

9. For a full rebuttal of the points made by Ntsaluba, see Nattrass (2001b).

10. Thanks to Alison Hickey for pointing out the implications for the budget process.

11. These points were echoed by all the responding provincial MECs for health in their accompanying affidavits. For example, the MECs for the Eastern Cape and Free State provinces argued that MTCTP (including training, testing and counselling) would cost more than the total budget allocated to AIDS. The figures presented were improbable and failed to take into account the savings to the state that would result from MTCTP.

12. The bulk of this money goes to life-skills training, and to the Eastern Cape, KwaZulu-Natal and the Northern Province. See Hickey (2002), Streak (2002) and Hickey and Ndlovu (2003) for a discussion of the allocation of AIDS-related funding through the budget.

13. It may be that the past failure of provincial governments to spend the available resource allocation for AIDS was more a function of the funding channel/ mechanism than of inadequate provincial management and skills (Hickey, private correspondence). If so, this provides even stronger grounds for optimism about spending delivery on AIDS in the future.

14. See, for example, the long list of obstacles recorded by David McCoy (a director of the Health Systems Trust) facing those wishing to implement MTCTP (*Mail and Guardian*, 4–10 May 2001).

15. The model can be downloaded from the website of the Actuarial Society of South Africa at www.assa.org.za/aidsmodel.asp. A user manual is also available as well as a spreadsheet containing summaries of the output and graphs.

16. The survey had a very low response rate – especially for the HIV testing – and appeared to have under-sampled people in informal settlements. Children under two years of age were not tested (and so recent cases of children infected with HIV by their mother were not picked up). Reported cases of sexually transmitted diseases were lower (and reported condom use higher) than those obtained through the demographic and health survey. Taken together, this indicates that those participating in the national survey were probably less vulnerable to HIV infection than the population at large.

17. See Johnson and Dorrington (2002) for a description of this model.

18. For a full description of the MTCTP intervention, see Geffen *et al.* (2003: 10–12) and Johnson and Dorrington (2002: 16–18).

19. The costing estimate in the appendix is slightly higher per child saved mainly because I assumed more additional deaths from substitute feeding than the ASSA2000 Interventions Model. If anything, I probably over-estimated the extra child deaths from substitute feeding, and the 'true' cost is probably closer to the ASSA2000 Interventions Model estimate than mine (R5,973).

4. Expanding an AIDS intervention to include HAART for all who need it

1. The ASSA2000 Interventions Model is the brainchild of Leigh Johnson and Rob Dorrington at the Centre for Actuarial Research (CARE) at the University of Cape Town. It is by far the most sophisticated demographic model in South Africa. See Van den Heever (2003) for a review of the ASSA models and other available demographic models.

2. This follows the clinical staging model used by the World Health Organisation. For a discussion of the empirical evidence and statistical modelling, see Johnson and Dorrington 2002, Appendix B.

3. This is drawn from European data (De Vincenzi 1994).

4. This is drawn from Ugandan data (Gray *et al.* 1998; Gray *et al.* 2001).

5. In a 2002 South Africa household survey, it was found that of those who admitted to having at least one STD diagnosed in the last month (2.3% of the sample), 39.9% were HIV-positive (as opposed to 13% among those with no diagnosed STD), and of those who had sores/ulcers on genitals in the past three months, 40.2% were HIV-positive (as opposed to the 13.3% who were HIV-positive with no such condition reported) (Shisana and Simbayi 2002: 55). Such data, however, does not prove that the presence of STDs makes a person more likely to be infected with HIV, because STDs and HIV cluster in the same populations. Nevertheless, there is international evidence that even after controlling for factors like behaviour and biological co-factors, the presence of STDs results in higher risk of HIV transmission (Corbett *et al.* 2002: 2179–80).

6. This may be an over-estimate because (*inter alia*) it does not take into account that people with symptomatic STDs are less likely to have sex.

7. Costs include drugs and time spent by medical personnel. One in six patients is assumed to be treated by a doctor rather than a nurse. Time spent treating women is assumed to be 20% higher than that for men, and 20% of cases are assumed to be misdiagnosed.

8. This is broadly consistent with findings from the 2001 South African national HIV prevalence survey. According to Shisana and Simbayi, 'among HIV-positive respondents who were sexually active in the previous year, awareness of serostatus was significantly associated with condom use at last intercourse, but that such relationship with condom use was not observed amongst HIV-negative respondents' (2002: 64).

9. This cost calculation includes the cost of personnel time, and of the Rapid HIV test (and Smartcheck confirmatory tests for those who test HIV-positive using the Rapid test). A factor is included to account for drop-out rates in the programme.

10. Zidovudine (AZT) and Stavudine (D4T) are examples of NRTIs, and Nevirapine

and Efavirenz are examples of NNRTIs. The other class of drug used in triple therapy is the protease inhibitor (e.g. Lopinavir and Nelfinavir).

11. The ASSA2000 Interventions Model assumes (following Rama and McLeod (2001)) that 17% of the population is covered by medical schemes and that 13% of births are to women covered by medical schemes.

12. The median period spent on first line treatment is slightly more than three years. The cost calculations presented here assume that first-line treatment costs R300 a month, and second-line treatment R450 a month. These prices are in line with the best prices available to the private sector in South Africa, but substantially more than the international best-price offers available, or of WHO pre-qualified generics (AIDS Law Project and Treatment Action Campaign 2003: 39). In other words, if the government undertook serious negotiations with the pharmaceutical companies, then cheaper drug regimens than the ones used in this study would be available.

13. The model assumes no change in the first- and second-line drug regimen. It does not, in other words, deal explicitly with the problem of drug resistance – although the additional care factor accommodates this to some extent. While drug resistance is often cited as a reason for not introducing HAART, Farmer et al. (2001: 406–7) point out that this is less of a problem with triple therapy combinations (as assumed in the ASSA2000 Interventions Model) than it is with monotherapy. And, as Harries et al. (2001) argue, irregular and unregulated access to antiretrovirals (which is currently the case in most of Africa) is more likely to generate resistant strains of HIV than a properly implemented national HAART programme. Drug regimens, even in a carefully managed national health intervention, will certainly have to change over time in response to resistance. Resistance is to be expected; the challenge is to manage it well.

14. The additional infrastructure cost includes a co-ordinator per site, office expenses for the co-ordinator, technical assistance costs and counselling rooms for the intervention sites. The public education cost covers community meetings, the employment of educators, and the purchase of materials. These are all based on information from MTCTP sites (mainly from Khayelitsha). The cost of providing condoms as part of a VCT intervention is also included in this line item.

15. For example, the annual hospitalisation cost of a child with AIDS using the Baragwanath data was estimated at R18,000, whereas the cost estimate used in Chapter 3 (based on Western Cape data) was R13,300.

16. However, Texiera et al. (2003) argue that if the cost of ambulatory care is included along with the drugs needed to treat opportunistic infections, then the health costs rise to $2 billion – which results in HAART actually saving the health sector money.

17. Badri et al. (2002) have shown that putting patients on HAART reduced the incidence of tuberculosis associated with HIV-1 by more than 80%. A study in Haiti

likewise concluded that 'as elsewhere, patients receiving HAART are far less likely to require admission to hospital than are patients with untreated HIV disease' (Farmer *et al.* 2001: 405). But while patients on HAART will require less treatment, they will revert back to a stage of higher AIDS-related morbidity if they become resistant to HAART and are forced to stop the treatment. As illustrated in Figure 4.4, the ASSA2000 Interventions Model assumes that people do eventually get pushed out of the HAART programme – and once this happens (as shown in Table 4.4) they suffer the same morbidity patterns as people who never went on it. In other words, the modelled benefit in terms of lower morbidity associated with HAART is less than suggested by short-term studies of the impact of going onto HAART.

18. As Farmer *et al.* argue with respect to the conventional wisdom that we cannot afford HAART: 'Leaving aside all moral arguments, any economic logic that justifies as acceptable the orphaning of children is unlikely to be sound, since the cost to society, though difficult to tabulate, is far higher than the cost of prolonging parents' lives so that they can raise their own children' (2001: 408).

19. DALY refers to 'disability adjusted life year' and is discussed in Chapter 3.

20. Marseille *et al.* warn that the benefits of reduced viral load have to be balanced against longer life expectancy for people on HAART (and hence a longer sex life) – an issue that is of importance if people on HAART increase their risky sexual behaviour (2002: 1854). The ASSA2000 Interventions Model includes a parameter to model lower viral loads and assumes people remain sexually active (see Table 4.4). The impact of this, together with increasing access to VCT, results in a net preventive impact.

21. Note that the model does not assume any increase in the proportion of HIV-negative people seeking counselling as a result of HAART becoming available. As the existence of a HAART treatment programme is likely to result in more HIV-positive and HIV-negative people getting counselled, the ASSA2000 Interventions Model may well be under-estimating the beneficial impact of HAART on prevention.

22. This is for the upper-bound and lower-bound hospitalisation costs respectively.

23. Boulle *et al.* observe that South Africa's costly arms procurement process could 'potentially have covered the entire cost of an antiretroviral intervention' (2003: 296).

24. This discussion draws on the discussion between medical practitioners, members of NGOs and AIDS advocacy groups held at the Children's Institute, University of Cape Town, on 4 July 2003. I would like to thank all participants (especially Andrew Boulle, Nathan Geffen and Paula Proudlock) for ideas and comments.

25. Brazil has massively expanded the domestic production of antiretrovirals under voluntary licensing agreements. Between 1999 and 2001, the proportion of anti-retrovirals produced in Brazil rose from 47% (19% of government expenditure on

antiretrovirals) to 63% (43% of expenditure). The remainder was purchased on the international market (Galvao 2002: 1864). Brazil has threatened to engage in compulsory licensing (i.e. breaking patents) in order to force price concessions from pharmaceutical companies, but has not yet done this. The November 2001 decision by the World Trade Organisation to allow the use of compulsory licensing in cases of national public health emergencies has further strengthened Brazil's hand – as well as that of other middle-income developing countries (like South Africa) that have the industrial capability to produce antiretrovirals if necessary.

26. The manufacturer, Aspen Pharmacare, also has voluntary licensing agreements with Boehringer Ingelheim (for Nevirapine) and GlaxoSmithKline (for Zidovudine and Lamivudine).

27. When Brazil and Botswana introduced their national treatment programmes, the state was actively involved in the setting up and management of additional testing facilities (Galvao 2002; Ramotlhwa 2003).

28. These include the MSF programme in Khayelitsha, other pilot projects in Gugulethu, Groote Schuur Hospital, and the Red Cross Children's Hospital, and clinical trials (e.g. at Somerset Hospital and Tygerberg Hospital).

29. The data on disability grants is not good enough to determine which grants are for people living with AIDS. This low assumed take-up rate is probably reasonable given the stigmatisation attached to AIDS (which prevents people from disclosing their status in order to apply for the grant) and the fact that many people do not get tested or know v they are entitled to the grant.

30. The Fiscal and Financial Commission has warned that this figure may be an under-estimate, and that more AIDS-related disability grants are likely in the future (*Cape Times*, 16 May 2003).

31. Households with working members are predominantly in the top half of the income distribution – whereas those without any members in employment are among the poorest, and can be regarded as comprising a marginalised 'under-class' (Seekings 2000).

32. This is the broad measure of unemployment – i.e. it includes those who report that they want work and does not require that they also be searching actively for it. See trend unemployment data for the 1990s in Nattrass (2000: 74).

33. There are strong indications that inequality worsened during the 1990s as unemployment rose. According to census data, the Gini coefficient (a measure of inequality ranging from 0 to 10) increased by 1 point between 1991 and 1996 (Whiteford and Van Seventer 2000). Household survey data from KwaZulu-Natal reported an increase in the Gini coefficient of four points between 1993 and 1998 (Carter and May 1999) – as did data from the income and expenditure surveys of 1995 and 2000. According to the KwaZulu-Natal survey (which collected informa-

tion on the same households in 1993 and 1998), the proportion of poor households rose from 35% to 42% over the five-year period.

5. AIDS, HAART and behaviour change

1. http://www.thebody.com/cdc/unsafe199/unsafe1999.htm
2. Own analysis of the Khayelitsha-Mitchells Plain data set (available from the Centre for Social Science Research at the University of Cape Town).
3. A focus group study of young African men found evidence for this myth (Tillotson and Maharaj 2001: 94), as did Mapolisa (2001: 56) in his study of young men in Gugulethu (Cape Town).
4. Reported in *The Economist*, 19 April 2003.
5. As Preston-Whyte and Zondi (1991) explain, the 'fertility conundrum' acts as a barrier to safer sex because young women are under pressure to prove their fertility before marriage. See also Tillotson and Maharaj (2001).
6. See review of evidence in Eaton *et al.* (2003) and Wojcicki (2002).
7. A recent study of the relationship between sexual violence and HIV preventive behaviour in South Africa found no statistically significant link between sexual abuse and condom use, but found that 'gender is an important influence on HIV preventive practices and needs to be more strongly emphasised in prevention programmes' (Jewkes *et al.* 2003: 132).
8. High levels of information about AIDS were recorded in the 2002 national household survey (Shisana and Simbayi 2002) and in two surveys of young adults (LoveLife 2000; Rutenberg *et al.* 2001: 35), yet this does not seem to translate into an equivalent high level of safe sexual practices. See also Eaton *et al.* (2003: 151–7) for a review of the evidence for high levels of knowledge about AIDS in South Africa.

6. AIDS, economic growth and inequality in South Africa

1. Non-response was particularly high for whites, and for adults and youth living in rural areas and informal settlements.
2. This is supported to some extent by national survey data, which found that HIV prevalence was lower for those with tertiary education (Shisana and Simbayi 2002: 54). An announcement by Anglo American that HIV prevalence was growing among its senior managers indicates that these figures may well be higher (radio report on AM Live, 13 August 2003).
3. The recent national household survey estimated white HIV prevalence to be much higher, i.e. 6.2% (Shisana and Simbayi 2002: 46). However, as there are problems regarding bias in the sample – and given the fact that the 95% confidence interval for this estimate is 3.1–9.2% – one should not conclude that this higher estimate

of white HIV prevalence is necessarily superior to estimates derived from other data sources.

4. See summary of international econometric studies of the economic impact of AIDS in Barnett and Whiteside (2002: 286–7). Most studies show a decline in per capita income as a result of the AIDS pandemic.

5. There are other macroeconomic models, but these are not as empirically rigorous as the models discussed here. ABT Associates (2000: 49–50) conclude that AIDS is likely to increase per capita incomes – but they do so not on the basis of their own macroeconomic model, but rather by reviewing modelling work from the rest of Africa and modifying it to take into account factors specific to South Africa (such as high unemployment). Bell *et al.* (2003) produce a macroeconomic model that is primarily driven by prior theoretical assumptions and has a weak South African demographic and empirical economic base. It was not deemed relevant enough to discuss in full in this chapter, although its major implication – that the long-term impact of AIDS could be substantial through its effect on education and skills – is referred to later.

6. See article in *The Economist*, 8 February 2001.

7. According to a recent survey of AIDS-affected households in South Africa, 34% of household income is spent on health care by AIDS-affected households. This is dramatically higher than the national average (4%) (Johnson *et al.* 2002). This is consistent with a study from Tanzania that found that people with AIDS had higher medical expenditure (and were more likely to seek medical assistance) than those with other terminal illnesses (cited in Desmond *et al.* 2000: 42).

8. Samson found that livestock ownership was an important source of savings, and that livestock sales were used to finance education and funerals. However, households reporting AIDS symptoms were less likely than other households to have sold livestock in the previous year (2002a: 1165).

9. CADRE argues that this is 'at odds with research elsewhere which suggests that households cut back on durable consumption to maintain food intake' (2000b: 14). In this regard, however, CADRE misses the point that the overall impact on demand is a function not only of changes in expenditure patterns at the level of the individual household, but also a function of the allocation of income between households.

10. ING-Barings assumes that 'for every person with full-blown AIDS, four months of person year equivalent labour supply will be lost' (2000: 11).

11. Employers shoulder two thirds of the higher medical cost burden in the ING-Barings model, and half in the BER model. Both assume that half of this burden is subsequently passed onto consumers. As regards indirect effects (i.e. lower productivity, increased turnover, recruitment costs, etc.) the BER model assumes

that productivity of infected workers is reduced by 40% (thus lowering the effective labour supply) and that this burden is shared between firms and consumers (BER 2001: 23). ING-Barings assumes no such additional reduction in the effective labour supply – hence the differences in projected trends for the labour force growth in the models (see Table 6.2).

12. CADRE has criticised this aspect of the ING-Barings model, describing the induced investment response as 'mechanistic' and failing to take into account the possibility that lower growth will undermine investor confidence – and hence will reduce investment (2000b: 15–16).

13. Arndt and Lewis assume that total factor productivity growth is reduced to one half of that in the no-AIDS scenario at the height of the epidemic. This is an attempt to capture more fully the harmful economic impact of hiring, training, absenteeism, work-force disruption, slower technological adaptation, etc. (2000: 872–4).

14. See Avetin and Huard (2000) for a clear exposition of this methodology as applied to three manufacturing firms in Côte d'Ivoire, and Barnett and Whiteside (2002) for a summary of studies of this nature.

15. Byrne reported that in a cement plant which had undertaken the voluntary saliva seroprevalence test among its employees, 79% of HIV-positive individuals were in the lower (predominantly unskilled) job bands (2001: 7). Sanders (2001: 16) reported that deaths in the Zimbabwe food manufacturing firm were all among the least skilled job categories.

16. See ILO 2000: 13–18 for a discussion of the impact of AIDS on enterprises in Africa. The impact will also depend on how many HIV-positive workers remain in employment. For example, research on the impact of AIDS on a South African colliery found that many workers who test HIV-positive leave immediately because they 'cannot handle the news' and 'just get up and run away' (Kennedy 2001: 10).

17. See also Thea et al.'s study of the impact of AIDS on 'company A' in South Africa (2000) and the review by Stevens (2001).

18. Morris and Cheevers report that the relatively low proportion of costs attributable to health care (11%) is similar to that found in a study of six companies in Kenya (2000: 7). They note that medical expenditure is not prominent in this population (i.e. the sugar mill) 'because of the public health system available' (2000: 943).

19. They use data on recruitment and training from a five-firm study in Botswana.

20. This is consistent with research from East Africa showing high costs associated with the disruption of production (ILO 2000: 14).

21. GEAR refers to the government's 'growth, employment and redistribution' policy framework.

22. See article in *Business Day*, 19 March 2002 (discussed in Chapter 2).

7. CONCLUSION

1. The 'People's Budget' is available on www.cosatu.org.za
2. See Seekings (2003a) for a discussion of the rival discourses.
3. In 1997, 5.5% of the labour force was employed in the government's Minimum Employment Plan (PEM) at wages equal to one third of the minimum wage. This rose to 8.5% in 1982 (Cortaza 1997: 237–9).
4. This assumes that each person works ten days a month, for R35 a day and that the wage bill absorbs 48% of the total resources required to run a national public works programme. The 48% wage bill figure was based on the average for the National Economic Forum job creation programme between 1992 and 1998.
5. The money could of course be raised through income tax rather than VAT. The discussion about taxation is presented here in terms of VAT simply to keep the argument simple.
6. Le Roux's (2002) proposed increase in VAT to fund a programme that costs R15 billion is larger than the VAT increase required to fund a PWP costing R22.8 billion. This is because the direct (or gross) costs of a BIG (R52 billion) are substantially larger than the net costs. By financing the BIG out of an increase in VAT, the tax system will 'claw back' the grant from richer people because they will end up paying more in expenditure taxes than they benefit from the grant. Le Roux also assumes increases in excise taxes.

References

Abdullah, F. 2003. 'Antiretroviral treatment: a provincial perspective'. Paper presented at the seminar on 'Scaling Up the Use of Antiretrovirals in the Public Health Sector: What are the Challenges?', the School of Public Health and the Perinatal HIV Research Unit, University of the Witwatersrand, 1 August.

ABT Associates 2000. *HIV/AIDS in South Africa – Implications for Investors.* Report prepared for J. P. Morgan, February.

ABT /Metropolitan 2000. *Demographic Impacts of HIV/AIDS in South Africa.* A study prepared for the Department of Finance by ABT Associates and the Metropolitan AIDS Research Unit, June.

AIDS Law Project and the Treatment Action Campaign 2003 (Belinda Beresford). *Hazel Tau and Others vs GlaxoSmithKline and Boehringer Ingelheim: A Report on the Excessive Pricing Complaint to South Africa's Competition Commission.* University of the Witwatersrand, Johannesburg.

Ainsworth, M. and M. Over 1994. 'AIDS and African Development'. *World Bank Research Observer*, 9(2).

Akeroyd, A. 1997. 'Socio-cultural aspects of AIDS in Africa: occupational and gender issues'. In G. Bond, J. Kreniske, I. Susser and J. Vincent (eds.), *AIDS in Africa and the Caribbean.* Boulder, Colorado: Westview Press.

Alexander, P. and T. Uys 2002. 'AIDS and sociology: current South African research'. *Society in Transition*, 33(3).

Allan, C. and X. Vitsha 2001. 'Comment to TAC on HIV/AIDS spending in Eastern Cape for 2000/2001 financial year'. Public Service Accountability Monitor, Rhodes University, Grahamstown.

Anand, S. and K. Hanson 1997. 'Disability-adjusted life years: a critical review'. *Journal of Health Economics*, 16: 685–702.

ANC 2002. 'Lend a caring hand of hope – statement of the National Executive Committee of the ANC'. Available on www.anc.org.za/ancdocs/pr/2002/pro32oa.html

Arndt, C. and J. Lewis 2000. 'The macro implications of HIV/AIDS in South Africa: a preliminary assessment'. *South African Journal of Economics*, August.

Avetin, L. and P. Huard 2000. 'The cost of AIDS to three manufacturing firms in Côte d'Ivoire'. *Journal of African Economies*, 9(2).

Badri, M., D. Wilson and R. Wood 2002. 'Effect of highly active antiretroviral therapy on incidence of tuberculosis in South Africa: a cohort study'. *The Lancet*, 359.

Barberton, N. 2000. 'Budgeting concerns around the care dependency grant and rough estimates of the cost of extending the grant to children affected by HIV/AIDS'. Revised input paper to the workshop 'Social Assistance Policy for Children with Disabilities and Chronic Illnesses', Child Health Policy Institute, Cape Town, May.

Barnett, T. and A. Whiteside 2002. *AIDS in*

the Twenty-First Century. New York: Palgrave Macmillan.

Baylies, C. and J. Bujra 2001. AIDS, Sexuality and Gender in Africa: Collective Strategies and Struggles in Tanzania and Zambia. London: Routledge.

Bell, C., S. Devarajan and H. Gersbach 2003. The Long-run Economic Costs of AIDS: Theory and Application to South Africa. Washington: World Bank.

Benatar, D. 2002. 'HIV and the hemi-nanny state'. The Lancet Infectious Diseases, 2 (July).

BER 2001. 'The Macro-economic impact of HIV/AIDS in South Africa'. Paper 10 (compiled by B. Smit, L. Visagie, and P. Laubscher), Bureau for Economic Research, University of Stellenbosch, 7 September.

Bhorat, H. 2002. 'A universal income grant scheme for South Africa: an empirical assessment'. Paper presented at the 9th International Congress of the Basic Income European Network, Geneva.

Bhorat, H. and J. Hodge 1999. 'Decomposing shifts in labour demand in South Africa'. South African Journal of Economics, 67(3): 348–80.

Bloom, D. and A. Mahal 1997. 'Does the AIDS epidemic threaten economic growth?' Journal of Econometrics, 9(2).

Bonnel, R. 2000. 'HIV/AIDS and economic growth: a global perspective'. The South African Journal of Economics, 65(5).

Booysen, F. 2002a. 'Poverty and health in Southern Africa: evidence from the demographic and health survey'. South African Journal of Economics, 70(2).

Booysen, F. 2002b. 'Financial responses of households in the Free State Province to HIV/AIDS-related morbidity and mortality'. South African Journal of Economics, 70(7).

Booysen, F. and J. Molelekoa 2001. 'The benefit to business of extending the working lives of HIV-positive employees: evidence from case studies in Bloemfontein and Welkom, Free State Province'. Paper presented at the 'International AIDS in Context' conference, University of the Witwatersrand, Johannesburg, 4–7 April.

Booysen, F., H. van Rensburg, M. Bachmann, M. O'Brien and F. Steyn 2001. 'The socio-economic impact of HIV/AIDS on households in South Africa: pilot study in Welkom and QwaQwa, Free State Province'. Draft interim report, Centre for Health Systems Research and Development, University of the Free State.

Booysen, F., H. van Rensburg, M. Bachmann, M. Engelbrecht and F. Steyn 2002. 'The Socio-economic impact of HIV/AIDS on households in South Africa: results of a Study in Welkom and QwaQwa, Free State Province'. AIDS Bulletin, 11(1).

Booysen, F., J. Geldenhuys and M. Marinkov 2003. 'The Impact of HIV/AIDS on the South African Economy: A Review of Current

Evidence'. Paper presented at the Trade and Industrial Policy Secretariat (TIPS) and the Development Policy Research Unit (DPRU) annual forum, Johannesburg.

Boulle, A. 2003. 'Capacity requirements for scaling up of antiretrovirals'. Paper presented at the seminar on 'Scaling Up the Use of Antiretrovirals in the Public Health Sector: What are the Challenges?', the School of Public Health and the Perinatal HIV Research Unit, University of the Witwatersrand, 1 August.

Boulle, A., C. Kenyon, J. Skordis and R. Wood 2002. 'Exploring the costs of a limited public sector antiretroviral treatment programme in South Africa'. *South African Medical Journal*, 92: 811–17.

Boulle, A., C. Kenyon and F. Abdullah 2003. 'A review of antiretroviral costing models in South Africa'. In J. Moatti, B. Coriat, Y. Souteyrand, T. Barnett, J. Dumoulin and Y. Flori (eds.), *Economics of AIDS and Access to HIV/AIDS Care in Developing Countries: Issues and Challenges*. Paris: ANRS.

Boyle, D. 2001. *The Tyranny of Numbers: Why Counting Can't Make us Happy*. London: Harper Collins.

Broomberg, J., M. Steinberg, P. Moasobe and G. Behr 1991. 'The economic impact of the AIDS pandemic in South Africa'. In *AIDS in South Africa: The Demographic and Economic Implications*. Johannesburg: Centre for Health Policy, University of the Witwatersrand.

Bundy, C. 1979. *The Rise and Fall of the South African Peasantry*. London: Heinemann.

Byrne, H. 2001. 'Reacting to the threat of AIDS: an exploratory case study of a South African firm'. Honours long paper, School of Economics, University of Cape Town. (Research supported by the Anglo American Chairman's Fund.)

CADRE (Centre for AIDS Development, Research and Evaluation) 2000a. *The Economic Impact of HIV/AIDS on South Africa and its Implications for Governance: A Bibliographic Review.* Compiled by CADRE (W. Parker, U. Kistner, S. Gelb, K. Kelly, M. O'Donovan and A. van Niekerk) on behalf of USAID through the Joint Centre for Political and Economic Studies. Johannesburg: CADRE.

CADRE 2000b. *The Economic Impact of HIV/AIDS on South Africa and its Implications for Governance: A Literature Review.* Johannesburg: CADRE.

Cameron, E. 2000. 'The deafening silence of AIDS'. Available on http://www.aids2000.com

Cameron, E. 2001. Opening address at the 'International AIDS in Context' conference, University of the Witwatersrand, Johannesburg, 4–7 April.

Cameron, E. 2003. 'The dead-hand of denialism'. An edited version of Cameron's Edward A. Smith Annual Lecture at Harvard Law School's Human Rights Programme. Printed in the *Mail and Guardian*, 17–24 April.

Campbell, C. 1998. 'The psychological context of HIV transmission on the gold mines: implications for HIV education programmes'. In B. Williams and C. Campbell (eds.), *HIV/AIDS Management in South Africa*. Johannesburg: Epidemiological Research Unit.

Carpenter, C. *et al.* 2000. 'Antiretroviral therapy in adults: updated recommendations of the International AIDS Society USA panel'. *Journal of the American Medical Association*, 283: 381–90.

Carter, M. and J. May 1999. 'One kind of freedom: poverty dynamics in post-apartheid South Africa'. Unpublished paper, University of Wisconsin, December.

Cherry, M. 2002. 'Botswana's AIDS laboratory squares up to HIV pandemic'. *Nature*, 418 (11 July).

CIDPC (Centre for Infectious Disease Prevention and Control, Canada) 2002. 'HIV infections among MSM in Canada'. *HIV/AIDS Epi Update*, April. Available on http://www.hc-sc.gc.ca

Cleary, S. and D. Ross 2002. 'The 1998–2001 legal struggle between the South African government and the international pharmaceutical industry: a game-theoretic analysis'. *Journal of Social, Political and Economic Studies*, 27: 445–94.

Coetzee, D. and A. Boulle 2003. 'Adherence: balancing ethics and equity, selection criteria and the role of DOT'. Paper presented at the seminar on 'Scaling Up the Use of Antiretrovirals in the Public Health Sector: What are the Challenges?', the School of Public Health and the Perinatal HIV Research Unit, University of the Witwatersrand, 1 August.

Cooper, F. 2002. *Africa Since 1940*. Cambridge: Cambridge University Press.

Corbett, E., R. Steketee, F. Oter Kuile, A. Latif, A. Kamali and R. Hayes 2002. 'HIV-1/AIDS and the control of other infectious diseases in Africa'. *The Lancet*, 359 (June 22).

Cortaza, R. 1997. 'Chile: the evolution and reform of the labour market'. In S. Edwards and N. Lustig (eds.), *Labor Markets in Latin America: Combining Social Protection with Market Flexibility*. Washington DC: Brookings Institution Press.

Cotton, M. F., H. S. Schaaf, E. Willemsen, M. van Veenendal, A. Janse van Rensburg and E. Janse van Rensburg 1998. 'The burden of mother-to-child transmission of HIV-1 disease in a "low" prevalence region – a five-year study of hospitalised children'. *The South African Journal of Epidemiology and Infection*, 13(2): 46–9.

Coutsoudis, A., K. Pillay, E. Spooner, L. Kuhn and H. Coovadia (for the South African Vitamin A Study Group) 1999. 'Influence of infant feeding patterns on the early mother to child transmission of HIV-1 in Durban, South Africa'. *The Lancet*, 354: 471–6.

Coutsoudis, A., K. Pillay, L. Kuhn, R. Spooner, W. Tsai and H. Coovadia (for the South African Vitamin A Study Group) 2001. 'Methods of feeding and transmission of HIV-1 from mothers to children by 15 months of age: prospective cohort study from Durban, South Africa'. *AIDS*, 15: 379–87.

Creese, A., K. Floyd, A. Alban and L. Guinness 2002. 'Cost-effectiveness of HIV/AIDS interventions in Africa: a systematic review of the evidence'. *The Lancet*, 359 (May 11).

Crewe, M. 1992. *AIDS in South Africa: Myth and Reality*. Penguin Books, London.

Crewe, M. 1998. 'The tangled webs of Virodene'. *AIDS Bulletin*, 5(2).

Crewe, M. 2000. 'South Africa: touched by the vengeance of AIDS: responses to the South African epidemic'. *South African Journal of International Affairs*, 7(1): 23–38.

Cross, C. 2001. 'Sinking deeper down: HIV/AIDS as an economic shock to rural households'. *Society in Transition*, 32(1).

Crothers, C. 2001. 'Social factors and HIV/AIDS in South Africa: a framework and summary'. *Society in Transition*, 32(1).

De Cock, K., D. Mbori-Ngacha and E. Marum 2002. 'Shadow on the continent: public health and HIV/AIDS in Africa in the 21st century'. *The Lancet*, 360 (July).

Decosas, J. 1998. 'Labour migration and HIV epidemics in Africa'. *AIDS Analysis Africa*, 9(2). Reprinted in E. Clarke, and K. Strachan (eds.), *Everybody's Business: The Enlightening Truth about AIDS*. Cape Town: Metropolitan.

Decosas, J. 2003. 'HIV prevention and treatment in South Africa: affordable and desirable'. *The Lancet*, 361 (April).

Department of Health 2001. *An Enhanced Response to HIV/AIDS and Tuberculosis in the Public Sector: Key Components and Funding Requirements, 2002/3–2004/5*. Pretoria: Department of Health.

Desmond, C., K. Michael and J. Gow 2000. 'The hidden battle: HIV/AIDS in the household and community'. *South African Journal of International Affairs*, 7(2).

De Vincenzi. I. (for the European Study Group on Heterosexual Transmission of HIV) 1994. 'A longitudinal study of human immunodeficiency virus transmission by heterosexual partners'. *New England Journal of Medicine*, 331: 341–6.

De Waal, A. 2003. 'How will HIV/AIDS transform African governance?' *African Affairs*, 102: 1–3.

De Waal, A. and J. Tumushabe 2003. *HIV/AIDS and Food Security in Africa: A Report for DFID*.

Dike, S. 2002. 'Research on the economic impact of HIV/AIDS in South Africa: review of methodology and lessons learned'. *South African Journal of Economics*, 70 (7).

Dladla, A., C. Hiner, E. Qwana and M. Lurie 2001. 'Speaking to rural women: the sexual partnerships of rural South African women whose partners are migrants'. *Society in Transition*, 32(1).

Dorrington, R. 2001. *The Demographic Impact of HIV/AIDS in South Africa by*

Province, Race and Class. Centre for Actuarial Research, University of Cape Town.

Dorrington, R., D. Bowne, D. Bradshaw, R. Laubscher and I. Timæus 2001. *The Impact of HIV/AIDS on Adult Mortality in South Africa.* Technical Burden of Disease Research Unit. Pretoria: Medical Research Council of South Africa, September. Available from http://www.mrc.ac.za/bod/index.htm

Dubois-Arber, F., F. Moreau-Gruet and A. Jeannin 2002. 'Men having sex with men and HIV/AIDS prevention in Switzerland'. *Euro Surveillance: European Communicable Disease Bulletin,* 7(2) (February).

Eaton, L., A. Flisher and L. Aaro 2003. 'Unsafe sexual behaviour in South African youth'. *Social Science and Medicine,* 56: 149–65.

Evian, C. 2000. 'Policy guidelines and recommendation for feeding of infants of HIV-positive mothers'. Prepared for the HIV Transmission and Breastfeeding Task Group. Available on www.doh.gov.za/aids/docs/feeding.html

Evian, C. 2003. 'An anonymous, unlinked HIV prevalence among a large workforce of agricultural/manufacturing employees in the Eastern (Lubombo) Swaziland region and comparison with the available local ante-natal HIV prevalence data'. Paper presented to the 'Demography and Socio-Economic' conference, Durban. Available on www.und.ac.za/und/heard/papers/conf

Farley, T., D. Buyse, P. Gaillard and J. Perriens 2000. 'Efficacy of antiretroviral regimens for prevention of mother to child transmission of HIV and some programmatic issues'. Background paper prepared for technical consultation on new data on the prevention of mother-to-child transmission of HIV and their policy implications. Geneva, October.

Farmer, P., F. Leandre, J. Mukherjee, M. Sidonise Claude, P. Nevil, M. Smith-Fawzi, S. Koenig, A. Castro, M. Becerra, J. Sachs, M. Attaran and J. Yong Kim 2001. 'Community-based approaches to HIV treatment in resource-poor settings'. *The Lancet,* 358 (August).

Fedderke, J. and M. Mariotti 2002. 'Changing labour market conditions in South Africa: a sectoral analysis of the period 1970–97'. *The South African Journal of Economics,* 70(5).

Forsyth, B. 2001. 'Reply to methods of feeding transmission of HIV-1 from mothers to children by 15 months of age: prospective cohort study from Durban, South Africa'. *AIDS,* 15: 1326–27.

Forsyth, B. and N. Nattrass 2002. 'A comment on "beyond informed choice" by Louise Kuhn'. *Social Dynamics,* 28(1): 155–161.

Forsythe, S. and M. Roberts 1994. 'Measuring the impact of HIV/AIDS in Africa's commercial sector: a Kenyan case study'. *AIDS Analysis Africa,* 4(5).

Fowler, M. and M. Newell 2000. 'Breastfeeding, HIV transmission and options in resource poor settings'.

Background paper prepared for Geneva UNAIDS/WHO/UNICEF meeting, October 11–13. Available on http://www.who.int/reproductive-health/rtis/MTCT/mtct_consultation_october_2000/consultation_documents/breastfeeding_and_HIV_in_resource_poor_settings/breastfeeding_and_HIV.en.html

Fox, M., S. Rosen, W. MacLeod, M. Wasunna, M. Bii, G. Foglia and J. Simon 2003. 'The impact of HIV/AIDS on labor productivity in Kenya'. Paper presented to the 'Demography and Socio-Economic' conference, Durban. Available on www.und.ac.za/und/heard/papers/conf

Freedberg, K. and Y. Yazdanpanah 2003. 'Cost-effectiveness of HIV therapies in resource-poor countries'. In J. Moatti, B. Coriat, Y. Souteyrand, T. Barnett, J. Dumoulin, and Y. Flori (eds.), *Economics of AIDS and Access to HIV/AIDS Care in Developing Countries: Issues and Challenges.* Paris: ANRS.

Galvao, J. 2002. 'Access to Antiretroviral drugs in Brazil'. *The Lancet*, 360 (7 December): 1862–5.

Geffen, N. 2000. 'Cost and cost-effectiveness of mother-to-child transmission prevention of HIV'. Briefing paper for the Treatment Action Campaign.

Geffen, N. 2002. 'A review of key research into the cost of highly-active anti-retroviral therapy'. TAC discussion document for the TAC/COSATU 'National HIV/AIDS Treatment Congress', June 2002.

Geffen, N., N. Nattrass and C. Raubenheimer 2003. 'The Cost of HIV/AIDS Prevention and Treatment Interventions'. CSSR Working Paper 29, Centre for Social Science Research, University of Cape Town. Available on www.uct.ac.za/depts/cssr

Ginwalla, S., A. Grant, J. Day, T. Dlova, S. Macintyre, R. Baggaley and G. Churchyard 2002. 'Use of UNAIDS tools to evaluate HIV voluntary counselling and testing services for mineworkers in South Africa'. *AIDS Care*, 14(5): 707–26.

Godfrey-Faussett, P., D. Maher, Y. Mukadi, P. Nunn, J. Perriens and M. Raviglione 2002. 'How human immunodeficiency virus voluntary testing can contribute to tuberculosis control'. *Bulletin of the World Health Organisation*, 80: 939–45.

Gow, J. and C. Desmond (eds.) 2002. *Impacts and Interventions: The HIV/AIDS Epidemic and the Children of South Africa.* Pietermaritzburg: University of Natal Press.

Gray, R., M. Wawer, D. Serwadda, N. Sewankambo, C. Li, F. Wabwire-Mangen, L. Paxton, N. Kiwanuka, G. Kigozi, J. Konde-Lule, T. Quinn, C. Gaydon and D. McNairn 1998. 'Population-based study of fertility of women with HIV-infection in Uganda'. *The Lancet*, 351: 98–103.

Gray, R., M. Wawer, R. Brookmeyer, D. Serwadda, N. Sewankambo, C. Li, F. Wabwire-Mangen, T. Lutalo, T. Cott and T. Quinn 2001. 'Probability of HIV-transmission per coital act in monogamous, heterosexual, HIV-1 discordant couples in Rakai, Uganda'. *The Lancet*, 357: 1149–53.

Grundlingh, L. 2001. 'A critical historical analysis of government responses to HIV/AIDS in South Africa as reported in the media, 1983–94'. Paper presented at the 'International AIDS in Context' conference, University of the Witwatersrand, Johannesburg, 4–7 April.

Haacker, M. 2001. *Providing Health Care to HIV Patients in Southern Africa.* IMF policy discussion paper, October. Available from mhaacker@imf.org

Habermas, J. 1974. *Theory and Practice.* London: Heinemann.

Haram, L. 2001. 'In sexual life women are hunters: AIDS and women who drain men's bodies. The case of the Meru of northern Tanzania'. *Society in Transition*, 32(1).

Harries, A., D. Nyangulu, N. Hargreaves, O. Kaluwa and F. Salaniponi 2001. 'Preventing antiretroviral anarchy in sub-Saharan Africa'. *The Lancet*, 358 (August).

Harrison, A., N. Xaba, P. Kunene and N. Ntuli 2001. 'Understanding young women's risk for HIV/AIDS: adolescent sexuality and vulnerability in rural KwaZulu-Natal'. *Society in Transition*, 32(1).

Harvard Consensus Statement 2001. Consensus statement on antiretroviral treatment for AIDS in poor countries. Individual members of Harvard University.

Hensher M. 2000. 'Confidential briefing: the costs and cost effectiveness of using Nevirapine or AZT for the prevention of mother to child transmission of HIV – current best estimates for South Africa'. Unpublished.

Hickey, A. 2002. 'HIV/AIDS spending policy and intergovernmental fiscal relations'. *The South African Journal of Economics*, 70(7).

Hickey, A. and N. Ndlovu 2003. 'What does budget 2003/4 allocate for HIV/AIDS?' *Budget Brief No. 127.* Cape Town: Research Unit on AIDS and Public Finance, IDASA.

HIV Management Services 1998. *Projections of Costs of Anti-Retroviral Interventions to Reduce Mother to Child Transmission of HIV in the South African Public Sector.* Technical Report to GlaxoWellcome, April.

Hunter, M. 2002. 'The masculinity of everyday sex: thinking beyond "Prostitution"'. *African Studies*, 61(1).

Ichharam, M. and L. Martin 2002. 'Explaining the low rate of HIV prevalence at RAU'. *Society in Transition*, 33(3).

IFAD (International Fund for Agricultural Development) 2001. Strategy Paper on HIV/AIDS for East and Southern Africa. IFAD, October.

ILO 2000. *HIV/AIDS in Africa: The Impact on the World of Work.* Geneva: International Labour Office.

ING-Barings 2000. *Economic Impact of AIDS in South Africa: A Dark Cloud on the Horizon.* Research conducted by Kristina Quattek, Global Research.

International Collaboration on HIV Optimism 2003. 'HIV treatments optimism among gay men: an international perspective'. *Journal of Acquired Immune Deficiency Syndromes*, 32: 545–50.

Jacobs, S. and R. Calland 2002. 'Thabo Mbeki: myth and context'. In S. Jacobs and R. Calland (eds.), *Thabo Mbeki's World*, Pietermaritzburg: University of Natal Press; and London: Zed Books.

Jewkes, R., J. Levin, A. Loveday and L. Penn-Kekana 2003. 'Gender inequalities, intimate partner violence and HIV preventive practices: findings of a South African cross-sectional study'. *Social Science and Medicine*, 56: 125–34.

Johnson, L. and R. Dorrington 2002. 'The demographic and epidemiological impact of HIV/AIDS treatment and prevention programmes: an evaluation based on the ASSA2000 model'. Paper presented at the 2002 conference of the Demographic Association of Southern Africa, Cape Town.

Johnson, S., G. Schierhout, M. Steinberg, B. Russell, K. Hall and J. Morgan 2002. 'Health needs and services for people with AIDS: the view from the household'. Draft paper for the *South African Health Review*.

Joint Health and Treasury Task Team (JHTTT) 2003. *Summary Report of the Joint Health and Treasury Task Team Charged with Examining Treatment Options to Supplement Comprehensive Care for HIV/AIDS in the Public Health Sector*. Released 1 August.

Available on www.gov.za/reports/2003/ttr010803.pdf

Jones, S. and C. Varga 2001. 'Bloodwise? Knowledge and attitudes pertaining to HIV and blood donation in Durban'. *Society in Transition*, 32(1).

J. P. Morgan 2001. *How to AIDS-Proof Your Consumer Portfolio*. Johannesburg: Fleming Martin Securities.

Kahn, J., E. Marseille and J. Saba 2002. 'Feeding strategies for children of HIV infected mothers: modeling the trade-off between HIV infection and non-HIV mortality'. In E. Kaplan and R. Brookmeyer (eds.), *Quantitative Evaluation of HIV Programs*. New Haven: Yale University Press.

Kaplinsky, R. 1995. 'Capital intensity in South African manufacturing and unemployment, 1972–90'. *World Development*, 23(2): 179–92.

Karim, S., Q. Karim, M. Adhikari, S. Cassol, M. Chersich, P. Cooper, A. Coovadia, H. Coovadia, M. Cotton, A. Coutsoudis, W. Hide, G. Hussey, G. Maartens, S. Madhi, D. Martin, J. Pettifor, N. Rollins, G. Sherman, S. Thula, M. Urban. S. Velaphi and C. Williamson 2002. 'Vertical HIV transmission in South Africa: translating research into policy practice'. *The Lancet*, 359 (March).

Karshenas, M. 2001. 'Agriculture and economic development in sub-Saharan Africa and Asia'. *Cambridge Journal of Economics*, 25: 315–42.

Karstaedt, A., T. Lee, A. Kinghorn and H. Schneider 1996. 'Care of HIV-infected adults at Baragwanath

Hospital, Soweto. Part 2: management and costs of inpatients'. *South African Medical Journal*, 86: 1490–3.

Kelly, K. and P. Ntlabati 2002. 'Early adolescent sex in South Africa: HIV intervention challenges'. *Social Dynamics*, 28(1): 42–63.

Kennedy, C. 2001. 'From the coal face: a study of the response of a South African colliery to the threat of AIDS'. Honours long paper, School of Economics, University of Cape Town. (Research supported by the Anglo American Chairman's Fund.)

Kennedy, C. 2002. 'From the coal face: a study of the response of a South African colliery to the threat of AIDS'. CSSR Working Paper 5, Centre for Social Science Research, University of Cape Town. Available on www.uct.ac.za/depts/cssr/pubs.html

Khoza, S. 2002. 'HIV, infant nutrition and health care: implications of the state's obligations in providing formula milk to prevent HIV transmission through breastfeeding'. Socio-economic Rights Project, Community Law Centre, University of the Western Cape.

Kinghorn, A. 1998. 'Interventions to reduce mother-to-child transmission in South Africa'. *AIDS Analysis Africa*, 8(5).

Kinghorn, A., T. Lee and A. Karstaedt 1996. 'Care of HIV-infected adults at Baragwanath Hospital, Soweto. Part 1: clinical management and costs of outpatient care'. *South African Medical Journal*, 86: 1484–9.

Kuhn, L. 2002a. 'Beyond informed choice: infant feeding dilemmas for women in low-resource communities of high HIV prevalence'. *Social Dynamics*, 28(1): 132–54.

Kuhn, L. 2002b. 'Rejoinder to Forsyth and Nattrass'. *Social Dynamics*, 28(1): 162–69.

Kuhn, L. and Z. Stein 1997. 'Infant survival, HIV infection and feeding alternatives in less-developed countries'. *American Journal of Public Health*, 87: 926–31.

Lane, P. 1998. 'Profits and wages in Ireland: 1987–1996'. *Journal of the Social and Statistical Society*, 27(5).

Laporte, A. 2002. 'A new decline in preventative behaviours among homosexual men: the role of highly active antiretroviral therapy'. *Euro Surveillance: European Communicable Disease Bulletin*, 7(2)(February).

LeBeau, D., T. Fox, H. Becker and P. Mufune 2001. 'Agencies and structures facilitating the transmission of HIV/AIDS in northern Namibia'. *Society in Transition*, 32(1).

Leclerc-Madlala. S. 1997. 'Infect one, infect all: Zulu youth response to the AIDS epidemic in South Africa'. *Medical Anthropology*, 17: 363–80.

Leclerc-Madlala, S. 2001. 'Demonising women in the era of AIDS: on the relationship between cultural constructions of both HIV/AIDS and femininity'. *Society in Transition*, 32(1).

Leclerc-Madlala, S. 2002. 'Youth, HIV/AIDS and the importance of sexual culture'. *Social Dynamics*, 28(1).

Leibbrandt, M., I. Woolard and H. Bhorat

2000. 'Understanding contemporary household inequality in South Africa'. *Studies in Economics and Econometrics*, 24(3).

Le Roux, P. 2002. 'Financing a universal income grant in South Africa'. *Social Dynamics*, 28(2).

Lipton, M. 1986. *Capitalism and Apartheid: South Africa, 1910–1986*. Aldershot: Wildwood House.

LoveLife 2000. *Hot Prospects, Cold Facts: Portrait of Young South Africa*. LoveLife in conjunction with the *Sunday Times*.

Lucchini, S., B. Cisse, S. Duran, M. de Cenival, C. Comiti, M. Gaudry and J. Moatti 2003. 'Decrease in prices of antiretroviral drugs for developing countries: from political "philanthropy" to regulated markets'. In J. Moatti, B. Coriat, Y. Souteyrand, T. Barnett, J. Dumoulin and Y. Flori (eds.), *Economics of AIDS and Access to HIV/AIDS Care in Developing Countries: Issues and Challenges*. Paris: ANRS.

Macheke, C. and C. Campbell 1998. 'Perceptions of HIV/AIDS on a Johannesburg gold mine'. *South African Journal of Psychology*, 28(3).

Mapolisa, S. 2001. 'Socio-cultural beliefs concerning sexual relations, sexually transmitted diseases and HIV/AIDS amongst young male clients at a Gugulethu STD clinic'. Master's thesis in social anthropology, University of Cape Town.

Marais, H. 2000. *To the Edge: AIDS Review 2000*. Pretoria: Centre for the Study of AIDS, University of Pretoria.

Marcus, T. 2001. 'Is there an HIV/AIDS demonstration effect? Findings from a longitudinal study of long distance truck drivers'. *Society in Transition*, 32(1).

Marcus, T. 2002. 'Kissing the cobra: sexuality and high risk in a generalised epidemic – a case study of white university students'. *African Journal of AIDS Research*, 1(1): 23–33.

Marseille E., J. G. Kahn and J. Saba 1998. 'Cost-effectiveness of antiviral drug therapy to reduce mother to child HIV transmission in sub-Saharan Africa'. *AIDS*, 12: 939–48.

Marseille E., J. G. Kahn, F. Mmiro, L. Guay, P. Musoke, M. G. Fowler and J. Brooks Jackson 1999. 'Cost effectiveness of single-dose Nevirapine regimen for mothers and babies to decrease vertical HIV-1 transmission in sub-Saharan Africa'. *The Lancet*, 354 (September).

Marseille, E., P. Hofmann and J. Kahn 2002. 'HIV Prevention before HAART in sub-Saharan Africa'. *The Lancet*, 359 (25 May).

Marshall, T. H. 1950. *Citizenship and Social Class*. Oxford: Oxford University Press.

Matisonn, H. and J. Seekings 2002. 'Welfare in wonderland? The politics of the basic income grant in South Africa, 1996–2002'. Paper presented at the DPRU/FES conference on 'Labour Markets and Poverty in South Africa', Johannesburg 22–24 October.

McCloskey, D. 1990. *If You're So Smart: The Narrative of Economic Expertise*.

Chicago: University of Chicago Press.

McCord, A. 2002. 'Public works as a response to labour market failure in South Africa'. CSSR Working Paper 19.

McCord, A. 2003. 'The Economics of employment generation'. Paper presented at a CSSR seminar, 6 March.

McFarlane, M., S. Bull and C. Rietmeijer 2000. 'The Internet as a newly emerging risk environment for sexually transmitted diseases'. *Journal of the American Medical Association*, 284(4).

McIntyre, J. 2003. 'HIV resistance'. Paper presented at the seminar on 'Scaling Up the Use of Antiretrovirals in the Public Health Sector: What are the Challenges?', the School of Public Health and the Perinatal HIV Research Unit, University of the Witwatersrand, 1 August.

McIntyre, J. and G. Gray 1999. 'Mother-to-child transmission of HIV: where to now?' *AIDS Bulletin*, 8(1).

McPherson, M., D. Hoover and D. Snodgrass 2000. 'The impact on economic growth in Africa of rising costs and labor productivity losses associated with HIV/AIDS'. CAER II Discussion Paper 79, Harvard Institute for International Development.

Merson, M., J. Dayton and K. O'Reilly 2000. 'Effectiveness of HIV prevention interventions in developing countries'. *AIDS*, 14 (suppl. 2): 68–84.

Meth, C. and R. Dias 2003. 'Increases in poverty in South Africa: 1999–2002'. Paper presented to the Trade and Industrial Policy Secretariat (TIPS) and the Development Policy Research

Unit (DPRU) annual forum, Johannesburg.

Meyer, J., M. Brown and D. Kaplan 2000. 'Assessing the South African brain drain: a statistical comparison'. Development Policy Research Unit Working Paper 0040, July. Available on www.uct.ac.za/depts/dpru

Michael, K. 2000. 'Unbelievable: AIDS reporting in the business press'. *AIDS Analysis Africa*, 10(4) (Dec. 1999/ Jan. 2000).

Mlongo, N. 2003. 'Feasibility and efficiency of HAART in resource poor settings'. Paper presented at the seminar on 'Scaling Up the Use of Antiretrovirals in the Public Health Sector: What are the Challenges?', the School of Public Health and the Perinatal HIV Research Unit, University of the Witwatersrand, 1 August.

Moatti, J., I. Doye, S. Hammer, P. Hale and M. Kazatchkine 2002. 'Antiretroviral treatment for HIV-infected adults and children: some evidence in favour of expanded diffusion'. In S. Forsythe (ed.), *State of the ART: AIDS and Economics*. The Policy Project.

Moatti, J., B. Coriat, Y. Souteyrand, T. Barnett, J. Dumoulin, and Y. Flori (eds.) 2003. *Economics of AIDS and Access to HIV/AIDS Care in Developing Countries: Issues and Challenges*. Paris: ANRS.

Mocroft, A., B. Ledergerber, C. Katlama, O. Kirk, P. Reiss, A. d'Arminio Monforte, B. Knysz, M. Dietrich,

A. Phillips and J. Lundgren (for the EuroSIDA study group) 2003. 'Decline in the AIDS and death rates in the EuroSIDA study: an observational study'. *The Lancet*, 362 (5 July): 22–9.

Morris, C., D. Burdge and E. Cheevers 2000. 'Economic impact of HIV infection in a cohort of male sugar mill workers in South Africa'. *The South African Journal of Economics*, 68(5): 933–46.

Morris, C. and E. Cheevers 2000. 'The direct costs of HIV/AIDS in a South African sugar mill'. *AIDS Analysis Africa*, 10(5) (Feb./March).

MSF 2003. *Providing Antiretroviral Therapy at Primary Health Care Clinics in Resource Poor Settings, Preliminary report May 2001–May 2002*. Medécins Sans Frontières and the School of Public Health and Primary Health Care, University of Cape Town.

Murray C. 1994. 'Quantifying the burden of disease: the technical basis for disability-adjusted life years'. *Bulletin of the World Health Organisation*, 72: 429–45.

Murray, C. and A. Acharya 1997. 'Understanding DALYs'. *Journal of Health Economics*, 16: 685–702.

Nattrass, N. 1996. 'Gambling on invest-ment: competing economic strategies in South Africa'. *Transformation*, 31: 25–42.

Nattrass, N. 1998. 'We cannot *not* afford AZT'. *Mail and Guardian*, 4–10 December. Available on http://www.sn.apc.org/wmail/issues/981204/news50.html

Nattrass, N. 2000. 'The debate about unemployment in the 1990s'. *Studies in Economics and Econometrics*, 24(3).

Nattrass., N. 2001a. Affidavit for the Treatment Action Campaign. Available on www.tac.org.za and on www.uct.ac.za/depts/cssr

Nattrass, N. 2001b. Answering affidavit (to Ntsaluba). Available on www.tac.org.za

Nattrass, N. 2001c. 'High productivity now: a critical review of South Africa's growth strategy'. *Transformation*, 45: 1–24.

Nattrass, N. 2002. 'Should youth unem-ployment be targeted as part of a comprehensive welfare policy in South Africa?' *Social Dynamics*, 28(2).

Nattrass, N. 2003a. 'The state of the economy: a crisis of employment'. In J. Daniel, A. Habib, and R. Southall (eds.), *The State of the Nation 2002/03*. Pretoria: Human Sciences Research Council.

Nattrass, N. 2003b. 'Unemployment and AIDS: the social-democratic challenge for South Africa'. Paper presented to the annual Trade and Industrial Policy Secretariat (TIPS) and Development Policy Research Unit (DPRU) annual forum, Johannesburg.

Nattrass, N. and J. Seekings 1997. 'Citizenship and welfare in South Africa: deracialisation and inequality in a labour-surplus economy'. *Canad-ian Journal of African Studies*, 31(3).

Nattrass, N. and J. Seekings 2001. 'Two nations: race and economic inequality in South Africa today'. *Daedalus*, 130(1).

NIAID (National Institute of Allergy and Infectious Diseases) 2000. 'The evidence that HIV causes AIDS'. National Institutes of Health, October. Available on www.niaid/ HIVcausesAIDS_10_00.html

Ntsaluba, A. 2001. Answering affidavit. Available on www.tac.org.za

O'Donnel, R. 2001. 'The future of social partnership in Ireland'. Discussion paper prepared for the National Competitiveness Council, May.

Oni, S., C. Obi, A. Okorie, D. Thabede and A. Jordaan 2002. 'The economic impact of HIV/AIDS on rural households in Limpopo Province'. *South African Journal of Economics*, 70(7).

Over, M. 1992. 'The macroeconomic impacts of AIDS in sub-Saharan Africa'. World Bank Technical Paper 3. Washington, DC: World Bank.

Page-Shafer, K., W. McFarland, R. Kohn, J. Klausner, M. Katz, D. Wohlfeiler, S. Gibson and the Stop AIDS Project 1999. 'Increases in unsafe sex and rectal gonorrhea among men who have sex with men – San Francisco, California, 1994–97'. *Morbidity and Mortality Weekly Report*. Centres for Disease Control and Prevention, 29 January. Available on http://www.thebody.com/ cdc/unsafe199/unsafe199.html

Paine, K., G. Hart, M. Jawo, S. Ceesay, M. Jallow, L. Morison, G. Walraven, K. McAdam and M. Shaw 2002. '"Before we were sleeping, now we are awake": preliminary evaluation of the stepping stones sexual health programme in the Gambia'. *African Journal of AIDS Research*, 1(1): 39–50.

Paltiel, D. 2000. 'Five Minutes with the Governor'. *Medical Decision Making*, 20(2).

Paltiel, D. and A. Stinnett 1998. 'Resource allocation and the funding of HIV prevention'. In D. R. Holtgrave (ed.), *Handbook of Economic Evaluation of HIV Prevention Programs*. New York: Plenum Press.

Parker, R. 2000. 'A summary discussion of the development of HIV/AIDS policy in Brazil'. *Urban Health and Development Bulletin*, 3(2). Medical Research Council of South Africa. Available on www.mrc.ac.za/ urbanbulletin/june2000

Pawinski, R., U. Lalloo, C. Jinabhai and R. Bobat 2002. 'Community-based approach to HIV treatment'. *The Lancet*, 359 (16 February).

Perez, K., A. Rodes and J. Casabona 2002. 'Monitoring HIV prevalence and behaviour of men who have sex with men in Barcelona, Spain'. *Euro Surveillance: European Communicable Disease Bulletin*, 7(2) (February).

Pool, R., S. Nyanzi and J. Whitworth 2001. 'Attitudes to voluntary counselling and testing for HIV among pregnant women in rural South-West Uganda'. *AIDS Care*, 13(5): 605–15.

Poku, N. 2002. 'Poverty, debt and Africa's HIV/AIDS crisis'. *International Affairs* 78(3): 531–46.

Preston-Whyte, E. and M. Zondi 1991. 'Adolescent sexuality and its implications for teenage pregnancy and

AIDS'. *Continuing Medical Education*, 9(11): 1389–94.

Quin, T. *et al.* 2000. 'Viral load and heterosexual transmission of human immunodeficiency virus type 1'. *The New England Journal of Medicine*, 342(13): 921–9.

Rama, P. and H. McLeod 2001. *An Historical Study of Trends in Medical Schemes in South Africa: 1974 to 1999*. CARE monograph 1, Centre for Actuarial Research, University of Cape Town.

Ramotlhwa, S. 2003. 'The Masa antiretroviral therapy in Botswana'. Paper presented at the seminar on 'Scaling Up the Use of Antiretrovirals in the Public Health Sector: What are the Challenges?', the School of Public Health and the Perinatal HIV Research Unit, University of the Witwatersrand, 1 August.

Rawls, J. 1971. *A Theory of Justice*. Oxford: Oxford University Press.

Rawls, J. 1993. *Political Liberalism*. New York: Columbia University Press.

Regensberg, L. 2001. 'Aid for AIDS: a disease management programme for HIV/AIDS'. Presentation to the actuarial science seminar, University of Cape Town, May.

Rhodes, M. 2001. 'The political economy of social pacts: "competitive corporatism" and European welfare reform'. In P. Pierson (ed.), *The New Politics of the Welfare State*. New York: Oxford University Press.

Richter, L., H. van Rooyen, V. Solomon, D. Griesel and K. Durrheim 2001.

'Putting HIV/AIDS counselling in South Africa in its place'. *Society in Transition*, 32(1).

Rorty, R. 1996. 'Moral universalism and economic triage'. Paper presented to the 1996 Philosophy Forum, UNESCO, Paris. Available on http://unesco.org/phiweb/txt/uk/2rpu/rort.html

Rosen, S., J. Simon and J. Vincent 2000. 'Care and treatment to extend the working lives of HIV-positive employees: calculating the benefits to business'. *South African Journal of Science*, 96 (June): 300–5.

Rosen, S. and J. Simon 2002. 'Shifting the burden of HIV/AIDS'. Centre for International Health, Boston University, USA. Paper available from sbrosen@bu.edu

Rothstein, B. 1998. *Just Institutions Matter: The Moral and Political Logic of the Universal Welfare State*. Cambridge: Cambridge University Press.

Rutenberg, N., C. Kehus-Alons, L. Brown, K. MacIntyre, A. Dallimore and C. Kaufman 2001. *Transitions to Adulthood in the Context of AIDS in South Africa. Report of Wave 1*. Horizons, University of Natal, Durban.

Samson, M. 2002a. 'HIV/AIDS and poverty in households with children suffering from malnutrition: the role of social security in Mount Frere'. *South African Journal of Economics*, 70(7).

Samson, M. 2002b. 'The social, economic and fiscal impact of a comprehensive social security reform for South Africa'. *Social Dynamics*, 28(2).

Sanders, C. 2001. 'The economic impact of HIV/AIDS on Zimbabwean food manufacturing firms'. Honours long paper, School of Economics, University of Cape Town. (Research supported by the Anglo American Chairman's Fund.)

Scanlon, T. 1982. 'Contractualism and utilitarianism'. In A. Sen (ed.), *Utilitarianism and Beyond.* Cambridge: Cambridge University Press.

Schneider, H. 2001. 'The AIDS impasse in South Africa as a struggle for symbolic power'. Paper presented at the 'International AIDS in Context' conference, University of the Witwatersrand, Johannesburg, 4–7 April.

Schneider, H. (ed.) 2003. *Scaling up the Use of Antiretrovirals in the Public Sector: What are the Challenges?* Proceedings of a seminar hosted by the School of Public Health and the Perinatal HIV Research Unit, University of the Witwatersrand, 1 August.

Schneider, H. and J. Stein 2001. 'Implementing AIDS policy in post-apartheid South Africa'. *Social Science and Medicine*, 52: 723–31.

Scott, J. 1976. *The Moral Economy of the Peasant: Rebellion and Subsistence in Southeast Asia.* New Haven: Yale University Press.

Seekings, J. 2000. 'Visions of society: peasants, workers and the unem-ployed in a changing South Africa'.

Studies in Economics and Econometrics, 24(3).

Seekings, J. 2003a. 'Providing for the poor: welfare and redistribution in South Africa'. Inaugural Lecture, University of Cape Town, 23 April.

Seekings, J. 2003b. 'Do South Africa's unemployed constitute an under-class?' CSSR Working Paper 32, Centre for Social Science Research, University of Cape Town. Available on www.uct.ac.za/depts/cssr

Seekings, J. 2003c. 'Unemployment and distributive justice in South Africa: some inconclusive evidence from Cape Town'. CSSR Working Paper 24, Centre for Social Science Research, University of Cape Town. Available on www.uct.ac.za/depts/cssr

Seekings, J. and N. Nattrass 2004 (forth-coming). *From Race to Class: Inequality during Apartheid and Post-Apartheid South Africa.* Yale University Press, New Haven.

Seekings, J., N. Nattrass and M. Leibbrandt 2003. *Inequality in Post-apartheid South Africa: Trends in the Distribution of Incomes and Opportunities and their Social and Political Implications.* Report for the Centre for Development and Enterprise, Johannesburg.

Shell, R. 1999. 'Halfway to the holocaust: the rapidity of the HIV/AIDS pandemic in South Africa and its social and economic consequences'. In *3rd Annual Population Conference*, 1. Pretoria: Centre for Epidemiological Research in Southern Africa.

Shisana, O. and L. Simbayi 2002. *South African National HIV Prevalence, Behavioural Risks and Mass Media*. Nelson Mandela/HSRC Study of HIV/AIDS. Pretoria: HSRC.

Sidley, W. 1953. 'The rational versus the reasonable'. *Philosophical Review*, 62 (October 1953): 554–60.

Simbi, T. and M. Aliber 2000. 'The agricultural employment crisis in South Africa'. Paper presented at the Trade and Industrial Policy Secretariat (TIPS) policy forum, Muldersdrift, September.

Simkins, C. 2003. 'Facing South Africa's social security challenge'. Unpublished paper, University of the Witwatersrand.

Skordis, J. 2000. 'Mother to child transmission of AIDS: what is the cost of doing nothing?' Paper presented at the 'Fourth International Conference on Healthcare Resource Allocation for HIV/AIDS and Other Life Threatening Illnesses', Cairo, October.

Skordis, J. and N. Nattrass 2002. 'Paying to waste lives: the cost-effectiveness of reducing mother-to-child transmission of HIV/AIDS in South Africa'. *Journal of Health Economics*, 21: 405–21.

Smith, A. 2000. 'HIV/AIDS in KwaZulu-Natal and South Africa'. *AIDS Analysis Africa* (Southern Africa Edition), 11(1).

Söderland N., K. Zwi, A. Kinghorn and G. Gray 1999. 'Prevention of vertical transmission of HIV: analysis of cost effectiveness of options available in South Africa'. *British Medical Journal*, 318 (19 June): 1650–56.

Sparks, A. 2003. *Beyond the Miracle: Inside the New South Africa*. Johannesburg and Cape Town: Jonathan Ball Publishers.

Steinberg, J. M., A. Kinghorn, N. Soderland, G. Schierhout and S. Conway 2000. 'HIV/AIDS: facts, figures and the future'. *South African Health Review 2000*. Durban: Health Systems Trust.

Steinberg, J., S. Johnson, G. Schierhout and D. Ndegwa 2002a. *A Survey of Households Impacted by HIV/AIDS in South Africa: What are the Priority Responses?* Report submitted to the Kaiser Family Foundation.

Steinberg, J., S. Johnson, G. Schierhout and D. Ndegwa 2002b. *Hitting Home: How Households Cope with the Impact of the HIV/AIDS Epidemic: A Survey of Households Affected by HIV/AIDS in South Africa*. Kaiser Family Foundation and the Health Systems Trust.

Stevens, M. 2001. *AIDS and the Workplace with a Specific Focus on Employee Benefits: Issues and Responses*. Centre for Health Policy, University of the Witwatersrand.

Stiglitz, J. 1998. 'More instruments and broader goals: moving towards the post-Washington consensus'. WIDER Annual Lecture 2, UNU World Institute for Development Economics Research, Helsinki.

Stillwaggon, E. 2002. 'HIV/AIDS in Africa: fertile terrain'. *The Journal of Development Studies*, 38(6): 1–22.

Stolte, G., N. Dukers, J. de Wit, H. Fennema and R. Coutinho 2002.

'A summary report from Amsterdam: increase in sexually transmitted diseases and risky sexual behaviour among homosexual men in relation to the introduction of new anti-HIV drugs'. *Euro Surveillance: European Communicable Disease Bulletin,* 7(2)(February).

Stover, J., N. Walker, G. Garnett, J. Salomon, K. Stanecki, P. Ghys, N. Grassly, R. Anderson and B. Schwartlander 2002. 'Can we reverse the HIV/AIDS pandemic with an expanded response?' *The Lancet,* 360 (6 July).

Streak, J. 2002. 'Mitigating the impacts with a focus on government responses'. In J. Gow and C. Desmond (eds.), *Impacts and Interventions: The HIV/AIDS Epidemic and the Children of South Africa.* Pietermaritzburg: University of Natal Press.

Stringer, J., D. Rouse, S. Vermund, R. Goldenberg, M. Sinkala and A. Stinnett 2000. 'Cost-effective use of Nevirapine to prevent vertical HIV transmission in sub-Saharan Africa'. *Journal of Acquired Immune Deficiency Syndromes,* 24: 369–77.

Strode, A. and K. Grant 2001. *The Role of Stigma and Discrimination in Increasing the Vulnerability of Children and Youth Infected with and Affected by HIV/AIDS.* Research Report commissioned by Save the Children (UK). Pretoria: Save the Children.

Sweat, M., S. Gregorich, G. Sangiwa, C. Furlonge, D. Balmer, C. Kamenga and O. Grinstead 2000. 'Cost-effectiveness of voluntary HIV-1 counselling and testing in reducing sexual transmission of HIV-1 in Kenya and Tanzania'. *The Lancet,* 356 (July).

Swift, J. 1729. *A Modest Proposal for Preventing the Children of Poor People in Ireland from being a Burden to their Parents or Country, and for Making them Beneficial to the Public.* Available on http://art-bin.com/art/omodest.html

TAC 2001. *TAC: An Overview.* Available on www.tac.org.za

TAC 2002. 'TAC's response to the Health Systems Trust report on mother-to-child-transmission prevention commissioned by the Department of Health'. Treatment Action Campaign, 27 February.

TAC 2003. *People's Docket.* Available on www.tac.org.za

Taylor Committee 2002. *Transforming the Present: Protecting the Future.* Report of the committee of inquiry into a comprehensive system of social security for South Africa. RP/53/2002. Pretoria: Government Printer.

Texiera, P., M. Vitoria and J. Barcarolo 2003. 'The Brazilian experience in providing universal access to anti-retroviral therapy'. In J. Moatti, B. Coriat, Y. Souteyrand, T. Barnett, J. Dumoulin and Y. Flori (eds.), *Economics of AIDS and Access to HIV/AIDS Care in Developing Countries: Issues and Challenges.* Paris: ANRS.

Thea, D., S. Rosen, J. Vincent, G. Singh and J. Simon 2000. 'Economic impact of HIV/AIDS in company A's workforce'. International AIDS Conference, Durban.

Thompson, E. P. 1963. *The Making of the English Working Class*. London: Victor Gollancz.

Tillotson, J. and P. Maharaj 2001. 'Barriers to HIV/AIDS protective behaviour among African adolescent males in township secondary schools in Durban, South Africa'. *Society in Transition*, 32(1).

Treasury 2003a. *2003 Budget Review*. National Treasury. Pretoria: Government Printer.

Treasury 2003b. *2003 Intergovernmental Fiscal Review*. National Treasury. Pretoria: Government Printer.

Trotter, G. 1993. 'Some reflections on the human capital approach to the analysis of the impact of AIDS on the South African economy'. In S. Cross and A. Whiteside, *Facing up to AIDS: The Socio-Economic Impact in Southern Africa*. London: Macmillan.

UNAIDS 1999a. *HIV/AIDS Prevention in the Context of New Therapies*.

UNAIDS 1999b. *Differences in HIV Spread in Four Sub-Saharan African Cities*. September. Summary is available on www.unaids.org/publications/documents/epidemiology/determinants/lusaka99.html

UNAIDS 2002a. *Report on the Global HIV/AIDS Epidemic*, July.

UNAIDS 2002b. *AIDS Epidemic Update*, December. Available on www.unaids.org

UNAIDS/WHO 2000. 'Joint UNAIDS/WHO press release:

preventing mother to child HIV transmission'. Available on www.who.int/reproductive-health

UNDP 1994. *1994 Human Development Report*. New York: United Nations Development Programme.

United Nations 2003. *East Africa: Feature – Traditional Culture Spreading AIDS*. Available on www.irinnews.org

Van den Heever, A. 2003. *Evaluation of the Sectoral Impact of HIV/AIDS in South Africa: A Methodological Review*. Pretoria: Human Sciences Research Council.

Van der Berg, S. and C. Bredenkamp 2002. 'Devising social security interventions for maximum poverty impact'. *Social Dynamics*, 28(2).

Van der Vliet, V. 2000. 'Established facts?' *AIDS Alert*, 93 (September).

Van der Vliet, V. 2001. 'AIDS: losing the "new struggle"'. *Daedalus*, 130(1).

VCTESG (Voluntary HIV-1 Counselling and Testing Efficacy Study Group) 2000. 'Efficacy of voluntary HIV-1 counselling and testing in individuals and couples in Kenya, Tanzania and Trinidad: a randomised trial'. *The Lancet*, 356: 103–12.

Vernazza, P. *et al.* 2000. 'Potent antiretroviral treatment of HIV infection results in suppression of the seminal shedding of HIV: the Swiss cohort study'. *Journal of Infectious Diseases*, 28: 117–21.

Walker, L. and L. Gilbert 2002. 'HIV/AIDS: South African women at risk'. *African Journal of AIDS Research*, 1(1): 75–85.

WCDH (Western Cape Department of Health) 1999. 'Programme for the prevention of mother to child transmission of HIV in Khayelitsha, Western Cape'. Presentation to the Provincial Health Restructuring Committee, 22 January.

Weeks, J. 1999. 'Stuck in low GEAR? Macroeconomic policy in South Africa, 1996–98'. *Cambridge Journal of Economics*, 23(4).

Weidle, P., T. Mastro, A. Grant, J. Nkengasong and D. Macharia 2002. 'HIV/AIDS treatment and HIV vaccines for Africa'. *The Lancet*, 359 (June).

Whiteford, A. and D. van Seventer 2000. 'South Africa's changing income distribution in the 1990s'. *Studies in Economics and Econometrics*, 24(3).

Whiteside, A. and C. Sunter 2000. *AIDS: The Challenge for South Africa*. Cape Town: Human and Rousseau.

Whiteside, A., R. Mattes, S. Willan and R. Manning 2002. 'Examining HIV/AIDS in Southern Africa through the eyes of ordinary Southern Africans'. CSSR Working Paper 11, Centre for Social Science Research, University of Cape Town. Available on www.uct.ac.za/depts/cssr

Wilkinson, D., K. Floyd and C. Gilks 2000. 'National and provincial estimated costs and cost effectiveness of a programme to reduce mother-to-child HIV transmission in South Africa'. *South African Medical Journal*, 90(8): 794–7.

Williams, B., D. Gilgen, C. Campbell, D. Taljaard and C. MacPhail 2000. *The Natural History of AIDS in South Africa: A Biomedical and Social Survey in Carltonville*. Johannesburg: CSIR (Council for Scientific and Industrial Research).

Wojcicki, J. 2002. 'She drank his money: survival sex and the problem of violence in taverns in Gauteng Province, South Africa'. *Medical Anthropology Quarterly*, 16(3).

Wojcicki, J. and J. Malala 2001. 'Condom use, power and HIV risk: sex workers bargain for survival in Hillbrow/ Joubert Park/Berea, Johannesburg'. *Social Science and Medicine*, 53(1): 99–121.

Wood, R. 2001. Affidavit for the Treatment Action Campaign. Available on www.tac.org.za

World Bank 2001. *World Development Report 2000/2001: Attacking Poverty*. Washington DC: World Bank.

World Health Organisation (WHO) 2000. 'New data on the prevention of mother to child transmission of HIV and their policy implications'. WHO technical consultation on behalf of the unfpa/unicef/who/unaid inter-agency task team on mother-to-child transmission of HIV. Geneva: WHO, October.

World Health Organisation 2002. 'Scaling up antiretroviral therapy in resource-limited settings: guidelines for a public health approach'. Available at http://www.who.int/hiv_aids

Index